Contents

KU-202-086

Preface

This book is an overview of fetal assessment. It is designed to provide the student midwife, and midwife, with easy reference to the main issues in this fast-growing and complex field.

CHAPTER ONE

Introduction

Interest in the well-being of the unborn child has always been in existence. Aristotle was aware of the progressive development of the fetus (Dryden, 1978) and was also interested in assessing the sex pre-delivery. He felt he could diagnose the sex of the fetus by the way it lay in the uterus or its mother's condition (Emery, 1973). This interest in the sex of the unborn baby continues to this day, with 'old wives' tales' living on, despite scientific evidence to the contrary. For example, studies have not confirmed links between the fetal heart rate and sex of the fetus (Steer, 1990).

However, in more modern times, interest in fetal assessment was inspired by a more serious intent – to reduce the mortality and morbidity of infants. Collections of data concerning perinatal deaths have been carried out since the early 1800s, although detailed analysis was not established until the work of Dugald Baird in the 1950s (Chamberlain, 1990). Fetal assessment in the United Kingdom could be said to have started in an organized fashion with the establishment of antenatal clinics, set up by Dr Janet Campbell in the 1920s (Chamberlain, 1990). Although the emphasis was very much on maternal well-being, it was assumed that improving the health of the mother would lead to a better outcome for the baby.

Ballantyne, in 1901, defined one of the three aims of antenatal care as the antenatal 'diagnosis of monsters'. However, although a multiple pregnancy can often be diagnosed by palpation, and the lack of movements and fetal heart tones can indicate fetal death, any more detailed diagnosis was not generally possible until the development of the use of ultrasound in obstetrics, pioneered by Professor Ian Donald in the 1950s (Proud, 1994).

Despite the rapid growth of fetal screening and diagnostic techniques, many traditional elements of fetal assessment continue. Fetal growth is routinely measured by abdominal palpation and clinicians' skills in predicting birth weights remain comparable to ultrasound estimations (see Chapter 2). Information of fetal position can likewise be obtained during palpation, and the outcome of labour influenced. However, the current easy access to ultrasound examination for confirmation of clinical findings may lead to a de-skilling of midwives and obstetricians in the future.

Another traditional part of fetal assessment is auscultation of the fetal heart, although its relevance in assessing fetal well-being is being questioned. Sharif and Whittle (1993) state the only benefit of routine auscultation is to reassure the mother her baby is alive. It is interesting to consider that women, who feel robust fetal movements, had probably no need of mechanical confirmation that their baby was alive, until habituated by professionals into the desirability of 'hearing' the fetal heart.

Present day routine antenatal care may now include methods of fetal screening, such as testing maternal serum for AFP levels and the 20 week anomaly scans. As procedures such as these are now so common, it is likely many women do not realize the implications of screening. For example, an AFP level in the accepted range or a 'clear' anomaly scan does not guarantee a 'perfect' baby. Also, ultrasound examination can be a diagnostic tool, as well as one used for screening, and women who do not want antenatal diagnosis may not realize this when attending their 'routine' scan.

More invasive procedures are now becoming almost routine for selected groups of the population. For many years women, on the basis of their age, have been offered amniocentesis for analysis of the fetus's chromosomes, it being accepted that the risk of abnormal fetal chromosomes increases with maternal age. However it is also true that most babies with chromosomal conditions are born to younger women, simply because they have more babies.

Therefore maternal serum screening (the triple test – see Chapter 5) was developed to find those younger women at risk, in order that they could be offered a diagnostic amniocentesis. It was also envisaged that older women who, after maternal serum screening, were demonstrated to have a reduced risk, would not wish an amniocentesis. However, there is evidence that women over 35 often choose to have an amniocentesis despite a low risk status (Green and Statham, 1993), and if this trend continues, many more amniocentesis will be carried out. The increasing identification by ultrasound of various 'markers' which may indicate a chromosomal abnormality (see Chapter 5) may also increase the number of amniocentesis done, as these women seek diagnoses. As many ultrasound 'markers' are not identified until the 20 week ultrasound, some women may want fetal blood sampling for karyotyping, rather than amniocentesis, to give a quicker result. This will lead to an increase in a potentially riskier procedure.

Women with post-term pregnancies are now often offered various fetal assessments to confirm the continued well-being of the fetus. The availability of these tests has no doubt reduced the number of unnecessary inductions, but most fetal assessment for post-term well-being is not yet of definite proven ability in confirming fetal health (see Chapter 4).

Despite the many techniques available to professionals, there is no sure way of guaranteeing the birth of a normal healthy baby. The major risks to the fetus are low birth weight, hypoxia and congenital abnormality.

Low birth weight due to premature birth can be serious for the infant, but although the outcome for even very premature infants has improved vastly over recent years, no way has yet been discovered of effectively predicting or preventing these births. Intrauterine growth retardation (IUGR) can be diagnosed in many cases during antenatal examinations (see Chapter 2) but again methods of prediction and prevention are still undiscovered. The role of the midwife in antenatal fetal assessment is especially important, as continuity of carer improves the potential for identifying a baby with sub-optimal growth. Much progress has been made in the diagnosis of chronic hypoxia, which is closely related to IUGR, and the possibilities exist of intervening by delivery for a fetus with chronic hypoxia before further deterioration in its condition. However intervention will also carry risks.

Congenital abnormalities can be increasingly accurately diagnosed, but in some cases more advanced techniques has provided many dilemmas for parents forced to make decisions about continuing a pregnancy where the outcome is unknown. Women may also need to make decisions about accepting invasive procedures for diagnosis on the basis of a numerical risk – when there is even a lack of consensus among professionals as to what is high or low risk (Garrett and Carlton, 1994).

Pregnancy will never be the same for women, as the availability and accuracy of fetal diagnosis grows. Women in the United Kingdom already have the right and ability to choose when to become pregnant and to abort a pregnancy they do not wish to have. However, the choices that face a woman with a wanted pregnancy are becoming ever more complex, and the role of the midwife is to be available with knowledge and support to assist a women during her decision-making.

CHAPTER TWO

Fetal Growth

'Growth is a product of the continuing and complex interaction of heredity and environment' (Tanner, 1989). The definition of a fetus is usually agreed to be from about ten weeks after the first day of a woman's last menstrual period (or eight weeks after conception) until birth. Prior to that, embryonic growth is mainly concerned with the development of organs. The head develops earlier than any other part of the fetal skeleton. At ten weeks gestation the fetus is about three centimetres long, with arms, legs, a beating heart and a nervous system that is beginning to show reflex responses.

More growth and development takes place during the 38 weeks of antenatal life than at any other comparable time in human life (Annis, 1978). The high rate of growth in the fetus is due to the fact that cells are still multiplying and maturing. The proportion of cells undergoing division in any tissue drops as the fetus ages. For example, it is thought that few new nerve and muscle cells appear after 30 weeks. The peak velocity of growth in weight is at about 34 weeks, and then begins to slow down. Up to 26 weeks most of the increase in weight is due to the storage of protein, as cells in the body are built up, but in the last ten weeks the fetus stores much energy in the form of fat. By 24 weeks the basis for fat tissue is laid down and from then fat accumulates - from 30-40 weeks fat increases from 30g to 430g (Tanner, 1989). At first the placenta grows quicker than the fetus, but after 30 weeks the fetus grows faster, and the placental: fetal size ratio falls.

The assessment of fetal growth is fundamental to monitoring well-being in antenatal care, and with good reason as low birth weight is a primary cause of perinatal mortality and morbidity. It is suggested that intrauterine growth retardation complicates from three to ten per cent of all pregnancies (Wagner, 1992).

Terms describing the weight and growth of the fetus/newborn are often used interchangeably and incorrectly.

Low birth weight (LBW)

A low birth weight baby is one who weighs less than 2500g at birth. This baby may be premature or small for gestational age (or both).

Small for gestational age (SGA) or small for dates (SFD)

This is a description of those babies (or fetuses) who weigh less than the tenth centile (i.e. their weight is within the lowest ten per cent when compared with the population of other babies of that gestation). Occasionally the fifth centile, or even the third centile is used as a description of SGA, but the tenth centile is by far the most common. SGA includes:

1. those babies who are normal 'small' babies, genetically determined to be small,
2. those babies with a congenital abnormality or environmental damage (for example, infection or fetal alcohol syndrome),
3. those babies who are intrauterine growth retarded.

Intrauterine growth retardation (IUGR)

This is a failure of growth which can be divided into two types.

Symmetrical growth retardation is when the whole fetus is small and can be diagnosed by identifying the same growth rate of the head circumference and the abdominal circumference. After investigation, these babies usually end up fitting into either groups 1 or 2, described above.

Asymmetrical intrauterine growth retardation is diagnosed when the rate of growth of the head circumference is normal but the growth of the abdominal circumference is below the normal velocity. This is caused mainly by a lack in the uteroplacental exchange system and is associated with maternal disease and/or malnutrition, or multiple pregnancy (Kenyon, 1994).

A fetus, or baby, may be IUGR but not SGA (less than the tenth centile). A term baby born weighing 3000g may have been genetically programmed to weigh (and have a head circumference corresponding to) 4000g. However, because of his/her birth weight, the growth retardation may go unrecognized.

Asymmetrical IUGR is an adaptation made by the fetus to balance demand to supply. By slowing growth he/she reduces their requirements and therefore can continue to exist on what is available. If necessary the fetus can take further adaptive actions, increasing perfusion of vital organs by redistributing cardiac output, responding to low oxygen levels by becoming polycythaemic and continuing to reduce growth by changing its hormone profiles. Changes in fetal blood gases, haematocrit, glucose and lactate levels are a late sign in IUGR (Clapp, 1989).

The 'brain-sparing' phenomenon of asymmetrical IUGR is limited. Brain weight has been shown to be reduced in both asymmetrical and symmetrical IUGR, but in asymmetrical IUGR the growth of the other organs are more severely retarded e.g. in asymmetrical IUGR the brain may have a reduction of 19-20 per cent, compared with 53 per cent reduction for the liver and 57 per cent for the spleen (Taylor, 1989).

A compromised fetus will have reduced blood flow to the renal system and this in turn results in reduced amniotic fluid. Oligohydramnios can therefore be a sign of a compromised fetus (Kenyon, 1994).

Asymmetrical IUGR can be diagnosed by serial ultrasound measurement of the head and abdominal circumferences at two weekly intervals. More frequent ultrasound assessment will not give an accurate picture (Proud, 1994). The well-being of the fetus can be assessed, with varying degrees of success, by biophysical profiles, liquor measurements and doppler blood flow studies (see Chapter 4).

Immediate consequences of IUGR may be meconium aspiration syndrome, operative delivery for fetal distress, stillbirth or neonatal death. A low birth weight baby may be separated from his or her mother if admission to a neonatal unit is necessary.

Neurological handicap is twice as common in SGA babies (Spencer, 1989). The fetus adapts to a progressive fall in oxygen levels from the placenta with a rise in haemoglobin concentration and increase in blood flow to the heart and brain, and this adaptation may be why 80 per cent of neurologically abnormal infants are delivered with normal blood gas values (Huisjes, 1980).

There is a theory that IUGR babies are 'programmed' into certain adult diseases, in particular heart disease (Barker, 1993). There seems some correlation between LBW and increased respiratory symptoms in children (Rona, Gulliford and Chinn, 1993) and an association between schizophrenia and obstetric complications at birth (most usually associated with IUGR) [O'Callaghan et al, 1992]. Cerebral palsy, long thought to be predominantly caused by birth injury, is now considered to be more usually associated with antenatal stresses on the fetus (Blair and Stanley, 1988).

Risk factors for IUGR

Many predisposing factors have been associated with IUGR. Maternal weight gain during pregnancy is a poor predictor of IUGR, but a low weight for height ratio at booking is associated with SFD's babies (Dawes and Grudzinskas, 1991).

Other risk factors include:
* history of premature or IUGR babies
* previous stillbirth or neonatal death
* maternal disease (e.g. existing cardiac, pulmonary or renal disease)
* pregnancy complications (e.g. pregnancy induced hypertension or antepartum haemorrhage)
* age (under 20 or over 35)
* low socio-economic group
* multiple pregnancy
* alcohol/substance abuse
* smoking.

Smoking in pregnancy is well known to be associated with intrauterine growth retardation, and it is suggested that ten cigarettes a day can lead to a birth weight reduction of 180g, and a 30 per cent increase in perinatal mortality (Tanner, 1989). There is evidence to suggest that the brand of cigarette smoked has an effect on the birth weight (Peacock et al, 1991). Non-smoking women living with smokers also appear to be susceptible to birth weight reductions (Martinez et al, 1994).

The role of the father in contributing to IUGR is being more widely examined at present. Regular alcohol drinking by the father prior to conception may reduce the birth weight of the newborn, and it is also suggested that exposure to toxins at work can lead to disease in the fetus/infant (Birth, 1992).

Mothers who suffered malnutrition in their childhood tend to have smaller babies. Studies have shown that if given nutritional supplements during pregnancy, they can increase the size of their babies, but not to the level of the babies of non-deprived mothers (Tanner, 1989).

There are some indications that IUGR can be caused by strenuous maternal activity impairing circulation to the uterus (Hytten, 1984) and therefore this suggests that heavy physical work or leisure activities may compromise fetal size.

Some studies have shown that increased stress factors independent of physical/medical conditions can lead to IUGR, as well as premature birth (Mutale et al, 1991; Wadhwa et al, 1993; Hedegaard et al, 1993).

Large for dates (LFD) babies, defined as those whose weights fall into the area above the 90th centile, are most often associated with maternal diabetes or maternal obesity, but some fetal anomalies can cause increased fetal growth.

Diagnosing intrauterine growth retardation

CLINICAL ASSESSMENT

Palpation of the growing fetus is a part of regular fetal assessment, but its degree of accuracy in identifying a fetus who has sub-optimal growth is questioned. There is certainly no doubt that accuracy can be vastly increased if there is continuity of carer throughout the antenatal period.

The most common way of assessing fetal growth by palpation is to compare the level of the fundus to a maternal landmark, assuming, for example, the fundus reaches the maternal umbilicus at 22-24 weeks, and the xiphisternum at 36 weeks. However, studies have shown maternal landmarks can be inconstant depending on the mother's torso size and shape (Royburt and Seidmann, 1990; Engstrom, 1988).

Measurement of the symphysis-fundal height by tape measure is now widely used and some authorities have quoted as much as 80 per cent success rate in identifying SGA fetuses with this method (Pearce and Campbell, 1987). There is however evidence that identification of the fundus during measurement is not always accurate (Engstrom, McFarlin and Sampson, 1993), and also that the tape measure is not an unbiased tool. Two studies have demonstrated that if the clinicians were aware of the gestation, this influenced their reading of the tape measure (Engstrom, Sittler and Swift, 1994; Rogers, Chan and Ho, 1992). Nevertheless, it appears that although the measurement of the symphysis-fundal height by tape measure is not ideal, it does improve on abdominal palpation alone in diagnosing IUGR fetuses (Stuart et al, 1989).

A simple measure that can increase accuracy in measurement of the fetal size is to ensure the woman passes urine before the abdominal examination. A full bladder has been demonstrated to cause a significant increase in measurement (Engstrom, Ostronga and Plass, 1989).

Besides assessing the size of the fetus in comparison with the weeks of gestation, during abdominal palpation clinicians often estimate the weight of a fetus, and it is accepted that an experienced midwife or doctor is usually as accurate as ultrasound examination in estimating birth weight (Neilson, 1990). This is especially true for a birth weight over 4000g (Chauhan et al, 1994) but a small study of fetuses ranging from 29-42 weeks gestation also demonstrated the accuracy of experienced midwives and obstetricians estimation of birth weight by palpation, in comparison with ultrasound examination (Hanretty, Neilson and Fleming, 1990).

Identification of oligohydramnious or polyhydramnios can also be made by a clinician during abdominal palpation, and appropriate investigations instigated to determine the cause. Those findings may be the first indication of an IUGR fetus, or one with a congenital abnormality.

An accurate abdominal palpation can be confounded by factors other than the fetus. The presence of fibroids may make the uterus seem large for dates, and an irregularly shaped uterus can cause the fetus to lay awkwardly and therefore make measurement difficult. Any factor which prevents the fetus entering the pelvis, such as a contracted pelvis, low-lying placenta or fibroids, or an ill-fitting presenting part, will influence the measurement of the fetus.

Any of the above factors can also cause an unstable lie of the fetus, and if this persists undiagnosed until labour, may of course cause fetal and/or maternal mortality or morbidity, through premature rupture of membranes, cord prolapse or obstructed labour.

Use of ultrasound in determining fetal age and growth

By six weeks gestation an embryonic sac can be seen on ultrasound, and a crown-rump length may be measured. The crown-rump length can give the most accurate assessment of gestational age (95 per cent of dates will be within five days accurate) but it is technically difficult as the degree of flexion of the fetus cannot be controlled. Therefore the biparietal diameter (measurement of the maximum transverse diameter between the parietal eminences) is more commonly used in dating scans, from about 12 weeks gestation. In second trimester ultrasounds this is usually correlated with another measurement (e.g. the femur length) to confirm the age (Proud, 1994) and there are now a range of normal values established for most fetal measurements (Neilson, 1990). After 28-30 weeks, an estimate of fetal age by ultrasound is not reliable as there is a wide range of fetal sizes and shapes by then.

An early 'dating' scan is becoming more widely used as part of routine antenatal care. It can be valuable for those uncertain of their last menstrual period, those who have a history of irregular menstruation, those who have been taking the combined oral contraceptive pill or those who have irregular bleeding (where an ultrasound scan can confirm viability or a missed abortion). It is estimated that as many as one quarter of women are uncertain of the date of their last menstrual period (Bennett et al, 1982).

A further emphasis on accurate dates has risen due to the increased use of maternal serum screening to determine the risk of fetal abnormality. Many centres include an early dating scan as part of the procedure in order to reduce the numbers of false positives due to 'wrong dates' or a multiple pregnancy.

It must always be remembered that a fetal anomaly can be detected on any ultrasound examination. For example during a dating scan a structural abnormality may be obvious, or if the BPD and femur length measurements do not correlate, a chromosomal abnormality may be suspected. In order to make an informed acceptance of a dating scan, the woman needs to be aware of this.

Before 24 weeks gestation, ultrasound scans can also provide baseline measurements for potential use in the third trimester if IUGR is suspected (Proud, 1994). If these are not available, serial ultrasound scans may be necessary to diagnose intrauterine growth retardation.

Assessment of sizes in a twin pregnancy can diagnose divergent growth, especially in twin to twin transfusion syndrome (Neilson, 1990) and therefore provide valuable information as to whether intervention may be necessary to preserve the vulnerable twin.

Fetal weight estimates by ultrasound can be calculated using established formulae based on various measurements (Hadlock, 1985). This may be done when considering delivery mode (for instance in a breech presentation), if considering induction for a maternal condition (e.g. PET, diabetes) or an IUGR fetus. A common use of fetal weight estimation is when premature labour has commenced (or needs to be induced), and an estimated fetal weight can give paediatricians necessary information when discussing likely outcomes with the parents prior to delivery. This information may also have an influence on the mode of delivery. It is especially important to correlate the estimated birth weight with gestation for premature fetuses, as a fetus who is premature and IUGR will have a different prognosis to one of the same gestation who is normally grown (Druzin, 1992).

Several studies confirm that establishing the gestational age of the fetus can reduce the induction rate for post term pregnancies (Bennett et al, 1982). It is interesting that studies done calculating the estimated delivery date (EDD) by either Naegele's Rule or obstetric wheels have proven unreliable in predicting the 'normal' 280 day pregnancy (McParland and Johnson, 1993). It would seem simply adding 280 days to the first day of the last menstrual period would give a more accurate result. Prolonged pregnancy is usually defined as after 42 completed weeks of pregnancy (294+ days). This affects about ten per cent of women, most commonly primiparas and those with a history of prolonged pregnancies, although maternal height and probably race also can be an influence (Saunders and Paterson, 1991). Although it is accepted that perinatal mortality rises after 294 days of pregnancy, there is no agreement as to what constitutes the best way of monitoring fetal well-being in prolonged pregnancy (Alfirevic and Walkinshaw, 1994).

A compromised fetus does not have to have a low birth weight, and conversely a low birth weight neonate is not always compromised (Tsang and Manning, 1994). However the early anticipation of those at risk of IUGR and the effective assessment and evaluation of fetal growth during pregnancy can surely help prevent not only the tragedy of stillbirth and neonatal death, but also reduce infant morbidity and perhaps also reduce long term childhood/adult health problems.

An audit carried out by Hepburn and Rosenberg in 1986 demonstrated that the maternity system was unable to identify antenatally more than one quarter of SGA babies. There is no evidence this figure has improved in recent years, and considering the potential IUGR has for lifelong consequences, this is an area which needs especial vigilance.

CHAPTER THREE

The Placenta

There is no doubt that the condition of the fetus is dependent on the integrity of the placenta and its ability to carry out exchanges efficiently with the maternal circulation. Over the years there have been many tests performed to try and assess the placenta and its function, as it was thought this would enable clinicians to evaluate fetal condition and also predict complications (Alexander et al, 1989). However, recently the emphasis on biochemical testing has given way to biophysical assessment, as this is currently deemed more reliable.

Examination of the placenta following birth is a routine part of the midwife's job. Inspection of placental structures by ultrasound is now possible antenatally but it seems that most structural deviations have no clinical significance (Fox, 1991). The exception to this may be an association between a circumvallate placenta and increased incidences of congenital abnormalities (Ladermacher et al, 1981). There could of course also be a risk to fetal well-being if there is a velamentous insertion of the cord, due to the potential for fetal blood vessel damage.

There have been studies looking at the placenta throughout pregnancy by ultrasound. Research has identified that by assessing the texture of the placenta, degrees of maturation can be established and there is an association between early placental maturation and perinatal problems (Proud, 1989). There has also been an association identified between premature maturation and smoking (Pinette, 1989).

Another ultrasound study of placentae scanned at two to four weekly intervals from 18-20 weeks gestation, identified a placental growth retardation at least three weeks before fetal complications such as intrauterine growth retardation, fetal distress or fetal death were diagnosed (Wolf, Oosting and Treffers, 1989).

Although most biochemical tests for fetal well-being have now been superseded by ultrasound and other biophysical tests in most centres, the following may still be in use.

Oestrogen

Oestriols form 90 per cent of the total oestrogens found in pregnancy and since the placenta produces oestriol in conjunction with the fetus, oestriol measurement has been seen as an assessment of placental/fetal well-being.

The assessment of oestriols can be made from a 24 hour urine collection or a serum specimen, the latter being considered less reliable. A low level of oestriol excretion can be associated with fetal intrauterine growth retardation and before the advent of biophysical profiles and doppler assessments, a falling level on serial estimations in late pregnancy was considered an indication for intervention.

Human placental lactogen (HPL)

Human placental lactogen is a polypeptide that is produced by the placenta in amounts regulated to the size of the placenta. HPL levels have been used as a test to assess fetal well-being, low levels being associated with intrauterine growth retardation. However, these tests are rarely done now as repeated studies have not shown the results to be reliably predictive of adverse perinatal outcomes (Gabbe, 1986).

Human chorionic gonadotrophin (HCG)

Human chorionic gonadotrophin is a glycoprotein secreted mainly by the trophoblast, but also by fetal tissues (Alexander et al, 1989). It is the basis for most pregnancy tests, and is used to help diagnose ectopic pregnancy and as part of the follow-up of in vitro fertilization.

HCG levels can diagnose a non-viable pregnancy in the presence of threatened abortion, but ultrasound is more usually used for this.

There may also be a correlation between abnormal HCG levels in late pregnancy and intrauterine growth retardation (Obiekwe and Chard, 1983) but, again, where ultrasound is available it provides a more accurate diagnosis.

Pregnancy-associated plasma protein A (PAPP-A)

Although PAPP-A has been found in the plasma of non-pregnant women (and men) its levels are much higher in pregnant women. At present it is unclear as to its source.

It has been reported that the levels of PAPP-A have been depressed in all women who seemed to have a viable pregnancy and then subsequently aborted (Westergaard et al, 1985). However it is difficult to see what clinical use can be made at present of this information. There may be a place for PAPP-A in diagnosing ectopic pregnancy, where some studies have reported abnormal PAPP-A levels (Grudzinskas, Westergaard and Teisner, 1986).

At present there seems to be potential for further research into the placenta, in the search for new and more reliable tests for fetal well-being. However, biochemical testing so far has been proven to be less efficient than biophysical tests such as ultrasound, doppler studies and cardiotocographs in the early detection or prediction of poor fetal outcomes (Arabin, 1995).

Therefore, where biophysical assessment is available, there currently seems no place for biochemical tests of the placenta except in an experimental capacity.

CHAPTER FOUR

Fetal Well-Being

Some women may begin pregnancy with a condition that requires careful surveillance of the fetus through every stage of its gestation, some women may have risk factors that could influence the fetus and therefore need increased attention, and some women will unexpectedly develop problems during their pregnancy that could compromise their fetus. The aim of antenatal fetal assessment is to ensure a term well-grown fetus, who is able to cope with the rigours of labour, but it is recognized that much birth asphyxia is not in those previously identified as a potential problem. In one study 50 per cent of 208 perinatal deaths had no identified risk factor (Low, Simpson and Ramsey, 1992). Those women who can be identified at booking as having a fetus at potential risk include:

- existing medical problems, for example renal or cardiac disease, epilepsy, essential hypertension, diabetes
- age (under 18 or over 35) and high parity
- smoking
- alcohol or drug abuse
- employment which entails predominantly standing in one position for more than three hours at a time as this has been reported as increasing the chances of premature labour (Teitelman et al, 1990).

During pregnancy conditions which arise that may compromise the fetus include:

- maternal infections (infection may cross the placenta to the fetus, or an accompanying maternal pyrexia may lead to spontaneous abortion or premature labour)
- multiple pregnancy – in some cases the outcome of a multifetal pregnancy can be improved with pregnancy reduction (Evans et al, 1993)
- placenta previa or unexplained antepartum haemorrhage

- recognized pregnancy complications. For example pregnancy-induced hypertension, polyhydramnios, gestational diabetes
- intrauterine growth retardation
- post-maturity – perinatal mortality rises in pregnancy after 42 weeks (Alfirevic and Walkinshaw, 1994).

Much routine antenatal care concerns assessing fetal well-being, and a midwife can obtain valuable information from a mother simply by discussing how the pregnancy feels to her. However, there are also many specific tests to consider.

Fetal movements

Fetal movements can usually first be felt by a primigravida at 18-20 weeks and by a multigravida at 16-18 weeks. Asking about the fetal movements is part of the midwife's antenatal check of a woman, but all midwives are aware that women can experience fetal activity differently – some are extremely aware of every movement and find them very uncomfortable, whereas some women are barely aware of any movements. It is important to discuss fetal movements with a mother so she becomes aware of her baby's pattern and realizes the importance of deviations. A reduction or cessation of fetal movements can signal an impending stillbirth.

Women often report more fetal movements at night, and this correlates with work showing that the diurnal motor activity in the fetus peaks at midnight (Patrick, 1982). There is also evidence that increased fetal movements may be associated with maternal emotion. For example in Italy following a volcanic eruption, many pregnant women attended hospital, reporting violent and continuous fetal movements followed by the absence of movements for six to eight hours (Visser et al, 1989). Smoking has been found to reduce fetal movements (Fisk and Rodeck, 1989).

Many centres give women, perceived to be at risk, or, in some cases, all women 'kick charts' late in the third trimester. The Cardiff 'count to ten' system is one of the most widely used. The woman contacts her midwife if she does not feel ten distinct movements in a set period of time (usually 12 hours). There have been some studies demonstrating that less than ten fetal movements in 12 hours is associated with fetal distress, fetal compromise and increased perinatal mortality (Fisk and Rodeck, 1989).

Cardiotocography (CTG)

There have not been any randomized controlled trials that have demonstrated a benefit from routine CTG monitoring for all women during pregnancy (Wheeler, 1991). However, continuous fetal heart cardiotocography for periods of about 30-60 minutes may be carried out in high risk women to aid in assessment of the fetus. This can be reassuring to the clinician, as a normal CTG trace can indicate a well oxygenated fetus at the time of the test in 99 per cent of cases. However, an abnormal CTG trace will probably only indicate hypoxia in 14 per cent of cases (Murphy et al, 1990).

Some studies have shown that routine antenatal CTGs in high risk pregnancies had no effect on perinatal morbidity or mortality and did not alter timing or mode of delivery, but did lead to fewer hospital admissions (Spencer, 1990).

The International Federation of Gynaecologists and Obstetricians issued guidelines in 1987 stating that antenatal CTGs should only be performed for clinical reasons and should not be interpreted in isolation from clinical signs (Spencer, 1990).

Although interpretation of a CTG trace may appear straightforward, a trace can sometimes be very difficult to decipher and research has shown that it can vary from one clinician to another (Mohide and Keirse, 1989). Interpretation of a CTG trace involves:

Fetal heart rate baseline

The fetal heart rate falls with advancing gestation. A normal baseline at the beginning of the third trimester is 120-160 beats per minute (bpm) but at term 110-150 bpm is acceptable (James, 1991). Fetal arrhythmias may indicate fetal heart disease, or have no clinical significance. A bradycardia may reflect a maternal condition (for example maternal systemic lupus erythematosus [SLE]), or may indicate fetal compromise. A tachycardia may also be related to maternal condition (for example, maternal pyrexia, thyroid disease or smoking) or may indicate fetal structural anomalies (James, 1993).

Variability

Variability is the variation in the baseline rate over one minute. The normal value is 5-15 bpm. The presence of variability is thought to reflect an intact pathway from the cerebral cortex, through the mid-brain to the vagus and conducting system of the heart. Therefore if cerebral tissue oxygenation is normal, the fetal heart should show normal variability (Druzin, 1992).

The fetus alternates between periods of 'sleep', diagnosed by reduced variability (and indicating reduced breathing movements, fewer body movements and lower fetal heart rate) and activity. These changes occur at intervals of about 20-40 minutes. The development of these two states is during the second trimester and is well established by 30 weeks gestation (Steer, 1990).

An unexplained 'sleeping' trace of more than 40 minutes can be a sinister sign.

In an effort to reduce the time spent attached to a CTG, there are many techniques midwives employ to stimulate a fetus with a sleep trace, to induce activity and obtain a reactive CTG trace with good variability. Studies have shown that many of these techniques, for example manual manipulation, glucose drinks, etc. are not effective – the only proven method is fetal vibro-acoustic stimulation (Hamner et al, 1993).

Accelerations

Accelerations (reactivity) is a temporary rise in the baseline of more than 15 bpm for 15 seconds or longer. This is usually in response to fetal or maternal movement. The normal value is at least two accelerations per 15-20 minutes.

The relationship between fetal movement and fetal heart rate accelerations depends on the integration of peripheral receptors, spinal cord, brain, autonomic nervous system and intact myocardium (Druzin, 1992).

Gestational age is correlated with accelerations and influences both the number and the size. At 28 weeks, ten per cent of normal fetuses have no accelerations of more than 15 bpm over the baseline (Pillai and James, 1990a).

Fetal movements, and therefore accelerations, can be influenced by maternal drugs (including smoking), hypoxia and acidosis.

Accelerations are regarded as a sign of fetal well-being and the relationship between the presence of accelerations and good perinatal outcomes has been widely demonstrated.

An example of difficulty in interpretation can arise when vigorous fetal movements can lead to a CTG showing large sustained accelerations with occasional returns to the baseline during pauses in activity. This trace could be misinterpreted as a 'tachycardia with decelerations' (Nijhuis, 1989).

Decelerations

Decelerations are a slowing of the fetal heart rate from the baseline of at least 15 bpm for at least 15 seconds. Decelerations are divided into:

- early (synchronous with a contraction and amplitude less than 40 bpm)
- late (the peak of the contraction and the lowest part of the deceleration have a lag time of more than 15 seconds)
- variable (described as an early deceleration with an amplitude greater than 40 bpm or variable in shape and occurring at variable times during contractions). Variable decelerations in the antenatal period are often associated with reduced amniotic fluid volume (Druzin, 1992).

A study described by Bekedam et al (1987) showed that fetuses diagnosed as intrauterine growth retarded and showing a decelerative CTG, had lower pO2 values at elective caesarean section than those with IUGR and no decelerations. The pH in the two groups were similar, which demonstrated that decelerations were associated with hypoxaemia, not acidaemia.

Even in the presence of accelerations, decelerations may indicate a poor perinatal outcome (Druzin, 1992). Decelerations unprovoked by contractions are a worrying sign.

Ultrasound

The role of ultrasound in assessing fetal well-being is common as part of the management or diagnosis of problems. Ultrasound is used to confirm the growth (or lack of it) in a fetus suspected of intrauterine growth retardation (see Chapter 2). It is also used to screen for or diagnose suspected abnormalities (see Chapters 5 and 6).

In the assessment of fetal well-being, especially in those babies diagnosed as intrauterine growth retarded, or in a post-term pregnancy, ultrasound forms part of other tests such as biophysical profiles.

Biophysical profile

As the central nervous system is among the tissues most sensitive to oxygen supply, the observation of this system can be an indirect indicator of fetal oxygenation (Tsang and Manning, 1992). The biophysical profile offers a structure to this observation.

A biophysical profile is a combination of assessments by ultrasound and cardiotocography. The biophysical variables include:

- fetal breathing movements
- gross body movement
- fetal tone
- qualitative measurement of amniotic fluid
- fetal heart trace.

Each of these variables is assessed and a numerical value is usually attached to the findings. The observation of normal fetal movements, tone and reactive heart rate, and at least one pocket of amniotic fluid measuring more than one centimetre in two perpendicular planes (see 'amniotic fluid measurement' below) will score '2' for each variable, totalling '10' – a fetus that could be defined at low risk for chronic asphyxia. Any abnormal observation would score '0' and a low total score may lead an obstetrician to suspect chronic asphyxia and consider immediate delivery (Gabbe, 1986).

A criticism of the biophysical profile is that the acute signs of fetal compromise (heart rate, fetal breathing movements, activity and tone) are given the same weight as chronic signs (amniotic fluid volume). It is suggested that a finding of oligohydramnios suggests an abnormal assessment, even if the other components are normal (Alfirevic and Neilson, 1993).

Biophysical scoring is not reliable in predicting fetal compromise in maternal diabetes as the pathological process may affect one or more of the biophysical parameters (James, 1993).

Amniotic fluid measurement

Many clinicians would not consider the one centimetre pocket of amniotic fluid, described above in biophysical profile, adequate, especially when assessing post-term pregnancies.

Normally amniotic fluid rises during pregnancy until approximately term, and then may drop slightly. The volume of amniotic fluid is the result of a balance between fluid production (primarily by fetal kidney and lung) and fluid removal (primarily by fetal swallowing). If the fetus is hypoxic, fetal renal and pulmonary perfusion drops, resulting in oligohydramnios developing over a period of days (Tsang and Manning, 1992).

The volume can be assessed subjectively, obtaining a general impression during abdominal palpation, or objectively by measurement on ultrasound.

There is research showing that the measurement of amniotic fluid using a four-quadrant amniotic fluid index (oligohydramnios is defined as less than or equal to five centimetres) is a better predictor of poor fetal outcome than a single largest pocket measurement (Youssef et al, 1993).

The presence of oligohydramnios may lead to increased risk of perinatal asphyxia and mortality. It may be associated with severe intrauterine growth retardation, renal abnormalities or an unrecognized rupture of membranes. Diagnosis can be difficult as the lack of amniotic fluid can lead to poor quality ultrasound images. However if doppler studies to assess uteroplacental waveforms are done, they are usually abnormal if the oligohydramnios is associated with intrauterine growth retardation (Hackett, Nicolaides and Campbell; 1987).

If necessary, amnio-infusion in the case of severe oligohydramnios can make the diagnosis easier, as ultrasound will be more effective and the fluid passing vaginally will confirm rupture of membranes. However this procedure could lead to infection or premature rupture of membranes (Catanzarite, 1993).

Fetal breathing movements

Observation of fetal breathing movements are used as part of a biophysical profile. The amount of time fetal breathing movements are present increases with gestational age until about 34 weeks, when there is a slight decrease until term (Pillai and James, 1990b). A healthy fetus has episodic, rapid and irregular breathing movements.

Fetal breathing movements rise in relationship to maternal glucose and caffeine (about two to three hours after a meal) and overnight during maternal sleep. They are reduced in the presence of alcohol and if the fetus is hypoxaemic or acidaemic (Richardson, 1989).

Doppler ultrasound studies

Doppler ultrasound is used to investigate uteroplacental and fetal blood flow. Doppler waveforms can be measured in the uterine artery and various fetal vessels, for example the umbilical artery, aorta, umbilical vein and cerebral and renal vessels. At present doppler studies on fetal umbilical artery waveforms are most commonly used and others are still mostly experimental. Continuous wave doppler compares the velocity of the blood during systole to that at the end of diastole (Proud, 1994).

Studies of umbilical artery flow velocity waveforms (FVW) reflect the placenta's vascular resistance and the perfusion of the feto-placental circulation. They do not show the fetal or uterine circulation (Dornan and Harper, 1994).

When a small-for-gestational-age fetus is identified, umbilical artery FVW may be able to predict those at risk. Studies have demonstrated that, according to fetal blood gases, umbilical artery FVW predicted fetal acidaemia better than biophysical profiles and CTGs (Challis, 1994).

It is thought that alteration in the fetal umbilical blood flow may occur in early fetal compromise. There is research assessing uncomplicated post-term pregnancies which demonstrates that those with abnormal doppler results were prone to need intervention for fetal distress (Anteby et al, 1994). Abnormal uterine artery FVW has been shown to be identified up to three weeks before signs of an abnormal CTG (McParland and Pearce, 1990).

Since maternal hypertension has been shown to cause abnormal umbilical artery waveforms (Trudinger, 1985) these women may benefit from routine doppler studies to diagnose early fetal compromise.

The absence of end diastolic frequencies in the fetal umbilical artery is a sign of fetal hypoxia (Nicholaides et al, 1988).

Doppler studies may also help to predict the severity of anaemia in red cell alloimmunized pregnancies by assessing such parameters as umbilical venous blood flow velocity and fetal aorta blood flow velocity. This could lead to fewer high-risk invasive tests and more accurate timing for intrauterine transfusion (Oepkes et al, 1994).

There may be a place in the future for doppler studies of the maternal uterine artery to be used as a screening test in order to diagnose the pathophysiological changes in early pregnancy. This can result in poor uteroplacental function and associated pregnancy complications such as pregnancy-induced hypertension, intrauterine growth retardation and placental abruption (Dornan and Harper, 1994).

Fetal blood sampling

Fetal blood sampling can be carried out under direct vision by fetoscopy or under ultrasound (cordocentesis). It can be carried out from about 16 weeks gestation and the usual site sampled is the umbilical vein about one centimetre from the placental cord insertion. Fetal blood can be used to diagnose a genetic condition (see Chapter 6) or a fetal infection (see Chapter 7).

Blood samples from hydropic fetuses can be diagnosed as non-immune or isoimmunized. In cases of isoimmunization, accurate haemocrit levels can be obtained and levels of anaemia can be assessed to determine the need for fetal transfusions.

A history of a previous baby affected with thrombocytopenia can be an indication for a fetal platelet count (Cherverak, 1992).

Fetal blood can also be used to assess acid base status to determine the optimum time for delivery, but doppler studies are more often used, being of less risk to the fetus.

Amniocentesis

Amniocentesis is primarily a diagnostic tool (see Chapter 6), but can also be used to assess fetal pulmonary maturity by testing the amniotic fluid for the lecithin:sphingomyelin ratio. A lecithin:sphingomyelin ratio of 2:1 indicates adequate surfactant in the fetal lungs and therefore respiratory distress syndrome of the newborn is unlikely to occur. This test is rarely done, as the risk of amniocentesis is unacceptable now the fetus can be assessed by biophysical means and the prognosis of premature babies is so improved.

At risk fetuses

The fetuses most commonly undergoing testing for well-being are those diagnosed as intrauterine growth retarded (IUGR) and those in a post-term pregnancy.

As discussed in Chapter 2, IUGR fetuses are at risk of asphyxia and there is evidence that the problems manifested at birth may not be due to the labour process, but exist antenatally (Nicolaides and Economides, 1990). Early diagnosis of problems will enable an IUGR fetus to be delivered at the optimum time.

Post-term pregnancies are also subject to increased assessments, due to the risk of adverse outcomes such as meconium aspiration syndrome, fetal distress or fetal acidosis. Commonly CTG, biophysical profiles and ultrasound estimation of amniotic fluid are used, and umbilical artery doppler studies are becoming more usual.

With the advent of wider availability of more sophisticated equipment and skilled operators, an expansion of tests for fetal well-being is inevitable.

CHAPTER FIVE

Fetal Screening and Genetic Counselling

Genetic disease can be divided into three main areas - single gene disorder, chromosomal abnormality and multifactorial conditions.

A pregnancy can be affected by genetic disease as a result of a family inheritance, a spontaneous mutation, maternal disease or age, or an environmental influence.

Single gene defects are a group containing many hundreds of conditions, most of them rare. However, also included are many of the most commonly screened for conditions such as the haemoglobinopathies.

This group also includes cystic fibrosis, the most common autosomal recessive disease in the North European caucasian population. The ability to screen for carrier status has been developed over recent years, but remains limited as only 70 per cent of cystic fibrosis is due to a specific mutation in an identified position on chromosome 7. The other 30 per cent can be caused by more than 100 different mutations (Meisner, 1993).

Chromosomal abnormalities are now relatively easy to diagnose by amniocentesis, and pre-diagnostic screening is increasingly available. The majority of chromosomal disorders have an extremely low risk of reoccurrence (Harper, 1981).

Multifactorial (or polygenic) conditions describe a large group of disorders which have a genetic component but have no clear pattern of Mendelian inheritance or chromosomal abnormality (Harper, 1981). They may arise from the combined effect of many influences: genetic, environmental or unknown. An example could be a fetal abnormality arising in the pregnancy of a mother with diabetes mellitus.

Preconception screening

For some women screening can start before pregnancy if they are diagnosed with a condition, or as a carrier of a condition, that could potentially affect a fetus in the future (for example sickle cell trait). It could be argued all these women should be offered preconception counselling. If a women and partner have a potential risk of an affected fetus in the future, it would seem to be an advantage to have information about possible outcomes of a pregnancy, the methods and implications of fetal diagnosis and choices that may be available, before the pregnancy occurs. By receiving and considering the information and choices available before pregnancy, making decisions during the antenatal period should be made easier.

For women with diabetes mellitus, good control of blood sugars at conception and during the early organogenesis period will reduce the chance of a fetal abnormality (Droste, 1993) and therefore these women can benefit greatly from preconception counselling and a planned pregnancy.

Many drugs have teratogenic effects, and those women needing regular medication need to discuss their drug regime before conception. While stopping a necessary medication may be dangerous, for example with epilepsy, often different drugs can be substituted which may have less potential effect on the fetus.

A low folic acid intake is known to be associated with an increased rate of fetal neural tube defects, and a folic acid supplement is now recommended for all women planning pregnancy (Department of Health, 1992).

Women with identified conditions may receive preconception screening, but the largest risk group seen before pregnancy is probably those counselled about future pregnancies after the birth of an affected baby, as this is often the first manifestation of a condition.

Maternal serum screening

Maternal serum screening is done routinely for some conditions in the antenatal period, and many women are first diagnosed as thalassaemia minor or sickle cell trait in pregnancy. These women need to be counselled and the results of their partner's test needs to be obtained before a prediction of the outcome for the fetus can be made. Where both partners carry the recessive gene, the couple may choose chorionic villus sampling (CVS) or fetal blood sampling (FBS) to obtain a fetal diagnosis.

Carrier status for other specific maternal or paternal genetic conditions (e.g. Tay-Sacks Disease) may also be tested for during pregnancy, but these are usually done before conception, as described above.

Alpha-fetoprotein (AFP)

AFP is an alpha globin produced by the fetus, and is present in the amniotic fluid, and in small amounts in the maternal blood. The levels in maternal blood can be most accurately assessed between 16 and 18 weeks. The level will be elevated in most pregnancies in which the fetus has a neural tube defect. It can also be elevated for other reasons such as wrong dates, multiple pregnancy, threatened abortion, intrauterine death or other anomalies (e.g. Turners syndrome or omphalocele). The cause of a raised AFP can also be unknown.

A major disadvantage of the test is the many false positives – it is estimated that for every 25 women having a single elevated AFP level, only one will eventually prove to have a child with a neural tube defect (Simpson, 1986). For this reason, women with a single elevated result may have a repeat test. If this is also elevated a detailed anomaly scan and, perhaps, an amniocentesis should be performed. Liquor AFP is a more accurate test than maternal serum. However, amniocentesis is now less frequently done following raised maternal serum AFP, as ultrasound is usually adequate to diagnose all neural tube defects (Kyle et al, 1994), or to identify other associated abnormalities, for example exompholos. However, if a condition such as exompholos is identified by ultrasound, an amniocentesis may be recommended for karyotyping, as this condition is often associated with chromosomal abnormality (Proud, 1994).

AFP screening was initially only used to screen for neural tube defects, a condition that accounts for approximately 50 per cent of congenital abnormalities diagnosed in the United Kingdom (Pearce, 1990). It is now also used as part of the 'triple test' screening.

Triple test (Barts Test)

The triple test consists of the results of serum alpha-fetoprotein, serum unconjugated oestriol and serum human chorionic gonadotrophin (hCG), taken together with the mother's age, to calculate the risk factor of a fetus with Down's Syndrome. This is done at 16 weeks gestation and since the normal serum values of human chorionic gonadotrophin, alpha-fetoprotein and oestriols vary with gestational age, it is extremely important to have accurate dates.

An ultrasound scan done prior to maternal serum screening, not only to confirm uncertain dates, but also to diagnose multiple pregnancy, will reduce the number of false positive results (Proud, 1994).

As the result is only a risk calculation, not a diagnosis, the 'high risk' woman must then decide whether to have an amniocentesis for a specific diagnosis. The usual cut off between high and low risk is 1:250, and it is suggested this will identify 60 per cent of affected fetuses (Chard and Macintosh, 1992). The actual odds of those with a positive screening being affected is 1 in 43 (Wald, Kennard and Densem, 1992).

In the constant search for the most reliable and cost-effective test, there are many variations of the triple test being researched. For example, the addition of measurements of urea resistant neutrophil alkaline phosphotase (Cuckle et al, 1990) or assessing human chorionic gonadotrophin in two parts (free α-hCG and free ß-hCG) [Wald et al, 1994]. The 'double test' assesses serum AFP and serum free beta-hCG.

Routine antenatal examinations

Midwives screen for abnormal fetal conditions during every antenatal visit, for example during the booking interview, through the tests they carry out and during their regular examinations throughout pregnancy. Many diagnoses arise from conditions first identified by a midwife.

Intrauterine growth retardation can be the first sign noted of a chromosome abnormality, and is a factor in many cases of fetal infection. Fetal growth is known to be clinically difficult to assess, and if a midwife suspects a reduction in growth, a referral for an ultrasound examination is usually appropriate. If growth reduction (or another finding such as microcephaly) is confirmed by serial ultrasounds, then further investigations may be offered.

The amount of liquor can also be significant. Polyhydramnios is associated with many abnormalities (for example oesophageal atresia, neural tube defects) as well as complicating normal pregnancies (for example, diabetes, multiple pregnancies). Oligohydramnios can be associated with renal abnormalities and can also cause compression deformities.

Some malpositions or malpresentations may be associated with abnormalities, for example hydrocephaly, and any fetal condition resulting in a lack of tone or deflexed head may cause a breech presentation or an unstable lie. A face presentation may be associated with anencephaly.

Now the majority of women have routine ultrasound examinations, many of these conditions will be identified before they result in assessable clinical signs. However, not all women accept the offer of routine ultrasound, and some conditions may only develop after the 20 week scan, so the midwife's skills of assessment will continue to be of importance.

Ultrasound

Ultrasound can be used as a screening or diagnostic tool (see Chapter 6). In the United Kingdom a routine ultrasound examination ('anomaly scan') is offered to all women at about 20 weeks gestation, in accordance with the recommendations of the Royal College of Obstetricians and Gynaecologists (RCOG, 1984). During this ultrasound, measurements of the fetus allow the estimated date of delivery to be confirmed, the site of the placenta is located and the fetus is examined for anomalies. However, the majority of abnormal findings will not be diagnostic in themselves, but identify a situation where amniocentesis or fetal blood sampling is necessary to obtain a definite diagnosis. Many anomalies identified will need referral to specialist units for specific diagnosis (for example, cardiac abnormalities) or rescanning at intervals to properly assess the situation (for example some renal tract anomalies). In some cases, the clinical significance of the findings is simply not known, and this is probably one of the hardest situations for the parents and the clinician.

Ultrasound can diagnose structural abnormalities such as neural tube defects or missing limbs. There are also many findings known as 'markers' (e.g. talipes, extra or missing digits or crossed fingers) which in isolation probably have no significance but if seen collectively may indicate a chromosomal defect (Proud, 1994). Nuchal skinfold thickness is seen by some authorities to be a marker for Down's Syndrome (Grandjean and Sarramon, 1995).

Choriod plexus cysts are a relatively common finding (about 25:1000) and often disappear by 24 weeks gestation (Gosden, Nicolaides and Whitting, 1994), especially if small and unilateral. However bilateral larger cysts may be associated with chromosomal abnormalities (in particular Trisomy 18).

Karyotyping is usually recommended if more than one marker is present (Proud, 1994).

Conditions which are identified, for example cardiac or renal anomalies, may also be associated with chromosomal abnormality.

There is some evidence that homozygous alpha-thalassaemia can be screened for in the second trimester by assessing placental thickness. At present this is usually only diagnosed by fetal blood sampling late in the second or in the third trimester after the development of hydrops (Ko et al, 1995).

As most of the abnormal findings during a routine ultrasound will not be diagnostic, there should always be a knowledgeable obstetrician, midwife or counsellor available during scanning sessions to discuss the findings, significance and possible further tests immediately an anomaly is identified. It is also of course necessary to have expert personnel available when a diagnosis is made, and in some cases a paediatrician may be the person with the most expertise in a particular condition.

Risk estimation

Women with a known inheritable condition or previously affected baby will, during genetic counselling, usually be given a risk estimation of a future (or present) pregnancy being affected. However over 90 per cent of all abnormalities happen in families with no previous history (Gosden, Nicolaides and Whitting, 1994). Maternal serum screening is also a way of giving all women a risk for their current pregnancy (albeit for a very limited number of conditions). A risk estimate is fundamentally a tool for decision making, and the decision each woman makes about the uptake of fetal diagnosis and what her actions will be following a positive diagnosis, is completely individual to her, and will reflect her physical, social, psychological, religious and cultural attributes and needs, as well as her personality.

Counselling that she receives should be non-directive, ensuring she has the facts to enable her to make a decision. However, it is accepted a counsellor's own views are difficult to conceal and even the presentation of facts and risk estimates can be directive (Harper, 1981).

A midwife's role is fundamentally enabling and supportive, ensuring the parents have access to specialized genetic counsellors if appropriate, and that they have an accurate understanding of screening procedures and their possible outcomes. The midwife may also need to provide emotional support following screening, while waiting for diagnostic results, and throughout the pregnancy and postnatal period if ambiguous results are identified or if the woman decides to continue with an affected pregnancy.

CHAPTER SIX

Fetal Diagnosis

A congenital abnormality is defined as a structural or functional fault that originates before birth and seriously interferes with the subsequent everyday life of the affected child (Dryden, 1978). There are three ways a fetal abnormality may be caused:

- chromosomal or genetic (either inherited or as damage)
- developmental damage (for example, by infection or a nutritional defect)
- damage during pregnancy (for example, hypoxia, an accident, prematurity or birth injury).

The field of fetal diagnosis has expanded greatly over the past ten years, and this shows no sign of slowing down. Diagnosis of some fetal abnormalities has become almost routine in many cases, and those with a microscopically visible chromosomal abnormality (e.g. Down's Syndrome being the most common) can usually be relatively easily and accurately diagnosed.

At present DNA analysis of chorionic tissue can diagnose several diseases (e.g. sickle cell disease, thalassaemia, haemophilia A and B) and the list is growing (Warren, 1990). Some inherited metabolic diseases can be diagnosed directly from amniotic fluid, although cultured cells are necessary for most. The diagnosis of single gene defects requires specific testing for the already diagnosed (usually following a previous affected baby) genetic problem, for which the fetus is known to be at risk.

There is no doubt that knowledge about, and methods of testing for, gene defects are growing rapidly. It is now theoretically possible to take a single cell, remove the DNA, and if there is knowledge of the location of the genome to be examined, enlarge that area to obtain enough DNA for gene probe analysis. As advances in gene mapping continue, it is not impossible that all single gene defects will one day be diagnosed by analysis of a single cell biopsy (Ferguson 1990, cited in Harris, 1991).

As further progress in this field is made, the number of women undergoing diagnostic tests for fetal abnormality will increase rapidly, especially as methods of screening for those considered 'at risk' expand and these women seek a definite diagnosis.

Ultrasound

Ultrasound is not only used as a screening tool, but also can be diagnostic in many instances.

Many structural abnormalities can be detected during ultrasound, and while some are pointers needing further investigation before a definite diagnosis can be made (e.g. reduced femur length could be present in several conditions), some findings are diagnostic in themselves (e.g. anencephaly).

Using a vaginal probe during ultrasound can result in visualization of the embryo earlier than by the usual abdominal transducer. This is usually only done in cases of family history of specific genetic abnormality when the parents want as early a diagnosis as possible (Proud, 1994).

It is estimated that a four chamber view of the fetal heart during ultrasound will detect approximately 95 per cent of all cardiac abnormalities. However, in many cases, even after a diagnosis of a fetal cardiac abnormality, the woman may need referral to a specialist ultrasound centre for another scan to determine the specific degree of abnormality and to receive a more detailed prognosis. For women with a family history or experience of cardiac abnormality, fetal echocardiography can detect structural heart disease accurately from early pregnancy (Sharland and Allan, 1990). Cardiac abnormalities are often present in other conditions (e.g. Down's Syndrome) and further investigation, such as chromosome analysis, may be necessary.

One of the most common areas for anomalies found by ultrasound is the fetal renal tract. The range of severity of the findings are vast. Bilateral renal agenesis is incompatible with life, but unilateral renal agenesis has a very good prognosis. The findings of renal cysts are common, and can vary in severity. A prognosis can often not be made as cysts may grow or regress during pregnancy (Fisk and Rodeck, 1990), although evidence of urine production is a good sign (Proud,

1994). Again, renal anomalies can often be a marker of another condition and may need further investigation. Additionally, some renal anomalies can only be fully investigated after the baby is born, and postnatal follow-up is important.

Chorionic villus sampling (CVS)

CVS is a sample from the chorion, taken via the cervix or transabdominally. In theory this can be done any time in pregnancy from seven weeks gestation, but the optimal time is 9-12 weeks (Warren, 1990).

Karyotyping can usually be obtained within 24-48 hours. Many metabolic disorders can be diagnosed by analysis of chorionic villi, either immediately or after cell culture. However, for those conditions with autosomal recessive inheritance, the maternal status must be established because contamination of the sample by maternal tissue may lead to a diagnostic error (Warren, 1990).

The advantages of CVS are the timing of results, which may be available in time for an early termination, if that is the mother's decision. There is also some evidence that CVS is perceived as less stressful and causes less anxiety than amniocentesis (Green, Statham and Snowdon, 1992), possibly due to being undertaken earlier in pregnancy.

Risks of CVS include miscarriage, infection and feto-maternal transfusion. The miscarriage rate following CVS is higher than that after amniocentesis. However this could be because the rate of spontaneous miscarriage at this time is greater than in later pregnancy. Recent studies have indicated that the previously reported link between CVS and limb abnormalities (Firth et al, 1994) may only occur in CVS undertaken before ten weeks gestation (Mastroiacovo et al, 1993).

There appears to be less risk of infection if the transabdominal route is used for CVS, rather than via the cervix (Fisk and Rodeck, 1989).

All Rhesus negative mothers are given anti-D immunoglobulin following any invasive procedure, in case of feto-maternal transfusion.

CVS cannot diagnose many common abnormalities and an anomaly ultrasound at the usual time is necessary to rule out such conditions as neural tube defects.

Amniocentesis

In the United Kingdom, amniocentesis is most usually carried out at 15-16 weeks gestation under ultrasound and strict aseptic conditions. A needle is inserted through the abdominal wall into the uterus and about 20 mls of amniotic fluid is withdrawn. There are usually a few viable cells in the fluid that can be cultured and in about two to three weeks these will have grown enough to analyse the chromosomes and to do metabolic studies. The cells can also be directly studied to confirm, for example, fetal sex or cell morphology.

Early amniocentesis, prior to 15 weeks, is practised widely in the USA and, with the improvement of ultrasound equipment and laboratory techniques, is becoming more common in the United Kingdom. The amount of amniotic fluid removed is less, the general rule being about one ml for each week of gestation.

The major advantage of early amniocentesis is to avoid late diagnosis of a fetal abnormality necessitating a late termination if appropriate.

In American studies there is a higher miscarriage rate in those amniocentesis done at or before 12 weeks, compared to those done after 15 weeks, but this may be because spontaneous miscarriage is more common in the first trimester.

Besides miscarriage, there is a risk of infection or premature rupture of membranes following amniocentesis. To prevent possible Rhesus isoimmunization of a Rhesus negative mother, anti-D immunoglobulin is given.

Some studies have been done into long term effects of amniocentesis on the baby/child. There has been a report of increased respiratory problems, but other studies have not demonstrated this. There has also been some indications of possible ear involvement during later aural development (Wapner, Johnson and Abbott, 1993).

Fetoscopy

A fetoscope can be inserted into the uterus transabdominally under ultrasound guidance. Examination of the fetus under direct vision can be done from about 15 weeks gestation, and skin or tissue samples can be obtained. Fetal biopsy can be undertaken, for example, if there is a familial history of a serious disorder such as epidermolysis bullosa, which can be diagnosed by fetal skin biopsy.

Risks of fetoscopy are spontaneous miscarriage, infection, feto-maternal transfusion (again, anti-D immunoglobulin will be given to all Rhesus negative mothers), and damage to the fetus during any biopsy procedure.

Fetal blood sampling

Fetal blood sampling can be carried out under direct vision by fetoscopy or under ultrasound guidance (cordocentesis). The usual site sampled is the umbilical vein about one centimetre from the placental cord insertion and about 20 mls of fetal blood is taken.

Indications for fetal blood sampling include a need for rapid karyotyping, perhaps following a failed amniocentesis or an ultrasound examination which showed possible markers of a chromosomal disorder, and a diagnosis can usually be available within about 48 hours.

A diagnosis of some conditions, such as haemoglobinopathies or coagulopathies can also be made following analysis of fetal blood.

The diagnosis of fetal infection may be made if IgM or viral particles are found in fetal blood, but there is currently no way of assessing the effect of the infection on the fetus.

Diagnosis of rhesusisoimmunization may be made, and this could be followed by on-going assessment of the fetal condition and treatment (see Chapter 4).

A diagnosis of chronic hypoxia can also be made after analysis of fetal blood, but other methods which carry less risk to the fetus, such as doppler studies, will probably be used (see Chapter 4).

At present few centres offer fetal blood sampling in pregnancy and a referral following preliminary findings is usually made as necessary.

There is a risk of miscarriage of about two to five per cent following fetal blood sampling, and also a risk of maternal haemorrhage or infection (Daker and Borrow, 1989). Cordocentesis may also be followed by transient bradycardia of the fetus, and a small bleed from the umbilical cord. Usually this has no clinical effect, but a persistent bradycardia may result in the necessity of immediate delivery (Chervenak, 1992).

A positive diagnosis

Following diagnosis of a fetal abnormality, in many cases the parents only have a choice of termination of the pregnancy or continuing until the birth of their affected baby. However, for some conditions there are some other choices available.

The field of fetal surgery is in its infancy but conditions such as hydrocephalus and bladder obstructions have been corrected during pregnancy with varying results (Proud, 1994). Bladder aspirations in some cases of obstructive uropathy and thoracocentesis to drain pleural infusion can take place either under ultrasound guidance or via a fetoscope. In the future there will no doubt be an expansion in the number of those conditions which can be helped surgically, and an improvement of outcomes will come with experience.

In some cases of fetal cardiac abnormality, drug treatment given to the mother can stabilize the fetal condition during pregnancy.

Some conditions, for example omphalocele or diaphragmatic hernia, have a good prognosis if the delivery mode and place is selected in order to obtain a birth which provides no further stress on the condition and ensures the baby receives immediate and appropriate treatment.

Fetal diagnosis of some abnormalities, in particular many cardiac and renal conditions, may lead to the newborn benefiting from early postnatal assessment and interventions, rather than waiting for symptoms to appear before investigations are carried out.

A particularly harrowing decision may need to be made by the parents of a multiple pregnancy in which, for example one fetus is diagnosed with an anomaly. If the abnormality diagnosed in one fetus is incompatible with life after birth, then nothing may be done unless the condition may compromise the other fetus (e.g. anacephaly may lead to polyhydramnios). If this is the case, or the abnormality is non-lethal and the parents choose, selective fetocide may be carried out by means of an injection of air into the umbilical cord or potassium chloride into the heart, of the affected fetus (Gibb and Greenough, 1992). There is a risk of miscarriage following this procedure.

Fetal diagnosis is a difficult area. The natural history of many minor abnormalities is unknown (Proud, 1994) and this can lead to much parental anxiety (and perhaps unnecessary terminations) about conditions with no clinical significance. There have been major advances lately in the number of gene defects that can be detected but the tests are time consuming and expensive and may be diverting limited resources away from areas of debatably greater need.

Simple identification of an abnormality cannot predict how an individual will be affected, for example some with cystic fibrosis are seriously ill their whole (short) life, while other are minimally affected (MacGregor, 1991).

However, there is no doubt that fetal diagnosis has altered the lives of parents at risk of having a baby with a known, perhaps familial, condition, who, without antenatal diagnosis may not have risked having a family. Now that there are many techniques for accurate fetal diagnosis, limiting these tests would seem an unethical denial of women's right to choose.

CHAPTER SEVEN

Fetal Infection

Although some amount of infection screening is routine for a pregnant woman, there is no routine screening for a fetus. The fetus is generally well served by two protective structures: the placenta and intact membranes. However, many infections can cross the placenta, in particular most viruses, but also some bacteria and protozoa (Fox, 1991). After rupture of the membranes (ROM), there is a danger of ascending infection.

Infections which cross the placenta can have varying consequences for the fetus, ranging from causing no discernible effect to fetal death. In general, the earlier in the gestation the infection occurs, the more severe the problem.

After ROM, some ascending infections, for example, Group B streptococcus, may have a disastrous affect on the baby, whereas others may respond easily to treatment and have no residual effect. Any woman with prolonged ROM should be screened for infection so, if necessary, prompt treatment of the neonate may limit any potential damage.

Many organisms, including those commonly found in vaginal flora (e.g. gardnerella vaginalis, ureaplasma urealyticum) can increase the risk of premature birth (McDonald et al, 1992) and it is usually the prematurity that puts the fetus/baby at risk.

It is thought that bacteria may start labour by direct effect on the amnion, as well as by other mechanisms (Bennett, 1988). However it is not possible to eradicate all pathogens from the vagina.

Risk groups

Women at risk from infection which may the affect the fetus/infant include those with a recent history of an infection, those with a permanent untreatable condition (e.g. herpes, HIV), or those with inadequate immunization (e.g. rubella). In certain areas some infections are endemic (e.g. malaria) which would pose a geographical risk factor.

Women who have suffered recurrent miscarriages or have had a previous perinatal death from unknown causes, may have an undiagnosed infection.

Some women have life styles which may make them vulnerable during pregnancy, for example a keen gardener may be at risk from toxoplasmosis, or a women working with young children may be at risk from chickenpox or parvovirus (B19).

All women are at risk of suffering a condition (e.g. influenza) involving a high pyrexia which could lead to fetal loss or damage, but those who are not in general good health (e.g. anaemic, malnourished) may be particularly vulnerable.

Any maternal infection has the potential of effecting fetal well-being, but the following are a summary of the most common.

Chlamydia trachomatis

Chlamydia is a bacterial infection which is increasing in both men and women. It is usually asymptomatic in women, but can cause premature ROM, premature labour, IUGR, stillbirth and eye or respiratory infection in the neonate (McGregor and French, 1991).

Cytomegalovirus (CMV)

Cytomegalovirus is a herpes virus and is spread throughout the body and can be passed on by many routes, including sexual activities. It is the most common cause of intrauterine infection, and the most common cause of congenital infection in the developed world, 1:300 births in the United Kingdom (Logan, 1990). However, although 50 per cent of fetuses may be infected, about 80 per cent of them will develop normally (Griffiths, 1991).

Cytomegalovirus can lay latent in maternal tissues and become reactivated during pregnancy (Stirrat, 1991). The presence of antibodies in the blood against CMV is indicative of infection, and virus specific IgM antibody is present in acute infections (Farr, 1988). The virus may also be cultured from maternal saliva or urine (Rowson et al, 1981), fetal blood or from amniotic fluid (Donner et al, 1994).

CMV is a slow growing virus and may not be detected for two to three weeks after the primary infection and then may take another two or three weeks until CMV excretion via the fetal kidneys is detectable in the amniotic fluid (Donner et al, 1994). There is evidence of possible false negative results when testing for CMV with amniotic fluid or fetal blood (Nicolini et al, 1994).

It is estimated that in industrialized countries 60-90 per cent of mothers have antibodies to CMV and although these antibodies do not protect against reactivation of the virus, they lessen the risk of fetal damage (Stray-Pedersen, 1993). However, primary maternal CMV infection can cause brain damage to the fetus during the first and second trimesters of pregnancy.

Other conditions which could occur in the baby include pneumonitis, neonatal hepatitis and various central nervous system disorders.

Gonorrhoea
Gonorrhoea is an infection by a gonococcus and is most usually sexually transmitted. Infected women may have a purulent discharge or dysuria, but many women are asymptomatic.

In early pregnancy, gonorrhoea may be associated with septic abortion. Later in pregnancy chorio-amnionitis may lead to premature ROM and preterm labour. Infection of the baby may occur during birth.

Group B streptococcus
Group B streptococcus is commonly found in the genital tract of symptomless women, and usually only becomes a problem during pregnancy, when it is associated with premature ROM and premature labour. Women in premature labour, or with prolonged ROM should be screened for Group B streptococcus as it is the most frequent cause of sepsis in neonates.

Treatment during pregnancy has not been shown to be effective but intrapartum antibiotics have offered a protection to the baby (Wang and Smaill, 1989). Several Scandinavian studies have concluded that douching with chlorhexidine can reduce the neonatal infection rate (Stray-Pedersen, 1993).

Hepatitis B virus

Hepatitis B is very common, with more than 200 million carriers in the world. The virus is found in saliva, semen, vaginal fluids and blood. It is usually transmitted by injection of infected blood or blood products.

Maternal serum is screened for HbsAg and then tested for 'e' antigens. If a woman is 'e' antigen positive, then there is a greater risk of maternal/fetal transmission and the baby will need treatment after birth (Griffiths, 1991).

There have been no teratogenic effects reported in fetuses, but an acute maternal attack in pregnancy can lead to a spontaneous abortion or premature labour.

Herpes simplex virus

Herpes is a virus that causes vesicular lesions, which can become latent and then reoccur, often at times of mental and physical stress (such as pregnancy). Some authorities believe that a primary infection during pregnancy can increase the risk of miscarriage or premature labour, and provide a small risk of congenital infection and congenital abnormalities (Watts, 1993).

Although there is some evidence that the virus can be transmitted to the fetus via the placenta (Logan, 1990), it is thought most cases of infection in the neonate are caused during birth.

At present, those with clinical evidence of active genital herpes at the time of delivery may be delivered by caesarean section, although this is more common in the case of a primary infection. There is some research that suggests treatment with acyclovir prior to the birth can reduce the reoccurrence of herpes at delivery and therefore decrease the need for caesarean section and the chance of neonatal infection (Stray-Pedersen, 1993).

Human immunodeficiency virus (HIV)

HIV is a retrovirus which is the causative organism of Acquired Immune Deficiency Syndrome (AIDS). It has been previously known as HTLVIII and LAV.

Two tests can be carried out for maternal diagnosis - the ELISA test (Enzyme Linked Immunosorbent Assay) and the Western Blot test. If both are done the result should be at least 99 per cent accurate.

At present there is no practical way of detecting the HIV status of a fetus and therefore care is directed towards reducing the chance of transmission. Studies have shown that maternal treatment with antiretroviral drugs during pregnancy and labour (in those HIV positive women previously untreated) can reduce the risk of HIV transmission (Connor, 1994). There is also evidence that transmission may be less likely following caesarean section, rather than vaginal delivery (Dunn et al, 1991). Care should also be taken to minimize invasive procedures such as CVS, FBS and application of fetal scalp electrodes, which may cause transmission of the virus to the fetus.

There is also a question of whether an HIV positive woman may be more prone to premature labour and an IUGR fetus, but this is controversial (Ryder, 1989).

Human parvovirus (B19) - (fifth disease)

Maternal parvovirus (B19) infection may be asymptomatic or cause a rash similar to rubella and arthralgia. Transmission to the fetus occurs in about one third of cases and about nine per cent of those infected may die, in association with hydrops fetalis (Best and Banatvala, 1990). There is no evidence that parvovirus (B19) causes congenital abnormalities in those infected infants who survive (Public Health Laboratory Working Party on Fifth Disease, 1990).

Listeriosis

Listeriosis is caused by a bacteria found widely throughout the environment. Advice is given to pregnant women to specifically avoid soft cheeses and patés, and to ensure cook-chill meals are well heated through.

Listeriosis can cause upper respiratory disease, septicaemia and encephalitic disease. Symptoms may be mild or severe, and include malaise, headache, fever, backache, and general influenza-like symptoms. Spontaneous abortion, preterm labour, stillbirth or meningitis (of mother or baby) could result.

Fetal mortality from listeriosis falls with rising gestational age (Ridgway, 1990). Diagnosis is made by culture of blood or cerebrospinal fluid.

Malaria

Malaria is usually caused by a bite from mosquitoes carrying the parasite Plasmodium falciparum, and is endemic in some parts of the world. Malarial attacks are common during pregnancy and can lead to miscarriage, premature labour, IUGR, stillbirth or neonatal death.

Rubella

Rubella during pregnancy may cause multiple fetal defects and sometimes intrauterine death. Although a comprehensive vaccination programme has been carried out in the United Kingdom for many years, all pregnant women are tested for rubella immunity at antenatal booking. Some women who have been previously vaccinated, and indeed previously tested as immune, have been known to become infected, or test as susceptible.

Symptoms of rubella can include a macular rash on the body, a low grade pyrexia and a general feeling of malaise. These symptoms can be so mild as to not be noticed at all by the woman. If a woman reports a contact with rubella, or complains of the above symptoms, a blood test is done.

Since blood for rubella serology takes 17 days to produce rubella IgG antibodies, if these are present before 17 days she is probably immune. If retesting after 17 days still shows no antibodies, this should be checked again four weeks after the contact.

If no antibodies are present, this should mean that there has been no infection (Griffiths, 1991). An infection can also be confirmed by the detection of rubella specific IgM antibodies, but these can show a false negative (Wang and Smaill, 1989). The rubella virus can also be detected with CVS (Terry et al, 1986).

Rubella can cause the loss of the pregnancy or the birth of a rubella-infected baby with various physical and mental anomalies. These include cardiac, eye and ear defects and mental and physical retardation. The fetus is most vulnerable up until 16 weeks, but the infection can cross the placenta at any gestation. An infected fetus after birth can be infectious for up to two years.

Syphilis

Syphilis, caused by the spirochaete treponema pallidum, is a sexually transmitted disease. At present it is rare in the United Kingdom, but there is some evidence that the incidence of syphilis in women of childbearing age is rising (Horner and Goldmeier, 1989). All women are screened antenatally because of the potential tragic effect on the fetus. Syphilis can cause loss of the pregnancy or the baby could be born with congenital syphilis, and may show signs of hepatosplenomegaly, anaemia, jaundice, rhinitis and central nervous system involvement.

Most of the symptoms of syphilis in the woman, such as the painless chancre in the primary stage and non specific rashes and lymph node enlargement in the secondary stage, may easily go unnoticed.

The diagnosis of syphilis can be made on scrapings of a lesion but serologic testing is more common.

Tests for syphilis include the treponema pallidum haemagglutination (TPHA), the rapid plasma reagin (RPR) and the venereal disease reference laboratory (VDRL). The Wasserman reaction (WR) has been largely replaced by the VDRL.

The RPR and VDRL tests are positive in 50-70 per cent of patients with primary lesions and almost 100 per cent of those with secondary or early latent syphilis (Ault and Faro, 1993).

It is possible to get true positive test results with yaws and pinta, and false positive results with malaria, leprosy, tuberculosis and glandular fever (Hurley, 1991). Those who abuse narcotics can also test as a false positive (Ault and Faro, 1993).

Syphilis is treated with antibiotics, penicillin G being the drug of choice. The longer the duration of the infection, the longer the course of treatment is necessary. Erythromycin does not cross the placenta, therefore does not prevent fetal congenital syphilis. Treatment in the third trimester may cause a pyrexial reaction (Jarisch-Herxheimer) which may predispose the woman to premature labour and fetal distress (Horner and Goldmeier, 1989).

RPR or VDRL titres should be repeated monthly until delivery, and these serial blood tests should show a decrease in titres if the treatment is effective. VDRL titres are generally lower than RPR, therefore these tests should not be used interchangeably when assessing the titre levels.

Toxoplasmosis

Toxoplasmosis is an infection caused by the parasite Toxoplasma gondii. It can be transmitted from domestic cat faeces, soil, raw meat and unpasteurized milk. The symptoms can be mild and influenza-like but most people have no symptoms at all. Infection can be confirmed by a rising titre (a positive titre of 1:500 or more is probably diagnostic) or the presence of specific IgM antibodies but interpretation of serological tests can be difficult.

Transmission to the fetus is less common, but more serious, during the first trimester (Wang and Smaill, 1989). Fetuses at risk are those whose mothers acquire a primary infection during pregnancy. Fetal diagnosis can be by analysis of amniotic fluid, fetal blood or placental tissue (Stray-Pederson, 1993). It is suggested that there is a rising risk of maternal transmission with increasing maternal age (Hohlfield et al, 1994).

There is some evidence that if infected women receive anti-parasitic treatment during pregnancy, this may offer a protective effect to the fetus (Berrebi et al, 1994).

Tuberculosis (TB)

TB in the United Kingdom, after years of being rare, is now a growing risk for the childbearing population. Transplacental infection is rare but does occur. Diagnosis of pulmonary TB is most commonly by X-ray, and the uterus can be protected with a lead shield during this procedure. TB may cause a miscarriage, or the woman may become so ill as to result in an IUGR fetus. Some drugs used in the treatment of TB have teratogenic effects.

Varicella-zoster (chickenpox) and herpes-zoster (shingles)

In the first and second trimester, maternal infection with varicella can occasionally cause fetal damage, including limb defects, microcephaly and cicatricial scarring (Best and Banatvala, 1990). Susceptible pregnant women can be given zoster immune globulin after exposure to chickenpox, but there is no evidence it prevents or modifies fetal infection or damage (Gilbert, 1993).

Maternal infection with varicella in late pregnancy may cause an infected fetus/neonate, depending on when the infection occurred. If the maternal rash appears 5-21 days before delivery, the infant is usually only mildly infected (probably due to the protective effect of maternal antibodies), but in those cases where the maternal rash appears from about four days pre-delivery to two days post-delivery, the infant may be severely infected (Logan, 1990). Treatment of potentially infected neonates by zoster immune globulin is recommended (Gilbert, 1993).

There has been no reported evidence of any effect on babies when their mothers suffered with shingles during pregnancy. Some healthy babies of mothers infected with chickenpox during pregnancy, did however contract shingles in their infancy.

In theory those fetuses who develop congenital abnormalities could be diagnosed by ultrasound in pregnancy, but in practice this may be a very late diagnosis, especially if the mother only contracted chickenpox in mid-second trimester. Also, the varicella virus may not activate in the fetus until some months after the primary infection. At present IgM or virus cultivation is not reliable - a negative result does not exclude infection, and evidence of intrauterine infection does not indicate fetal damage (Enders et al, 1994).

Diagnostic procedures

Many maternal infections can be diagnosed by maternal serum analysis, but this does not confirm an infection in the fetus, or identify damage even if the fetus is infected.

A fetal diagnosis of infection can sometimes be suspected on ultrasound examination (e.g. microcephaly/hydrops) or confirmed (e.g. limb deformities in the fetus of a woman following exposure to chickenpox).

Amniocentesis is sometimes used, but reliable tests on amniotic fluid are still being developed, although progress in this field is growing rapidly.

Fetal blood sampling can be carried out if there is evidence of maternal infection or ultrasonographic evidence in the fetus of potential infection. However, a positive result does not predict how the infection will affect the infant (Watts, 1993). A false negative result may also be possible, as a specific fetal IgM antibody may not appear in the fetal blood for some time (Miller, 1990).

The question has also arisen as to the possibility of infecting a previously uninfected fetus with maternal infection during an invasive procedure (Giorlandimo et al, 1994).

The two largest causes of perinatal death, and probably also infant morbidity, are congenital abnormality and prematurity. The leading part infection plays in both these conditions, underlines the importance of the subject.

CHAPTER EIGHT

Conclusion

If all fetal assessment involved risk-free testing, provided clear-cut answers and there were treatments available for any disorder found, there would be no controversy surrounding the subject. However, the reality is that the field of fetal assessment is growing so rapidly that new tests are available faster than society is able to evaluate the consequences, and it will be a long time, if ever, before many of the ethical dilemmas arising will be concluded.

Ultrasound assessment has been common in obstetrics for many years and is now regarded as a routine – and valuable – tool. The routine ultrasound scan is probably not one that causes many women anxiety. In fact, there is evidence that ultrasound is not viewed as a test at all, but as a chance to 'see' the baby (Green, Statham and Snowdon, 1992).

There is research that ultrasound can be of benefit psychologically, demonstrating that a group that could see the fetus on ultrasound felt more positive about the pregnancy and baby than a group that had the image shielded from them (Campbell, 1982). However there was no comparison with an unscanned group. There is also a suggestion that after early pregnancy bleeding, seeing a live fetus on ultrasound may improve the prognosis (Proud, 1994).

It is however likely that many, if not most, women do not perceive a routine ultrasound as a test which may not only diagnose a lethal abnormality in their baby, but also may identify a potential problem that may involve many further tests, and even then may not reach a meaningful diagnosis. Also, seeing the baby during an ultrasound and receiving the information that all the tests are within normal limits, may provide prospective parents with the assumption that a healthy baby is guaranteed.

Maternal serum screening (the 'triple/double test') is a relatively new test, but the availability is growing rapidly. Little work has been done at present on how women feel about receiving a 'high risk' result. Individuals will no doubt have varied responses but there are some indications that the attitudes of the carers are a large influence on how they cope (Newburn, 1993).

There is some evidence that women with false positive results and an unaffected child may remain anxious (Marteau et al, 1992). Women who have negative results after testing, and then have an abnormal baby have not yet been studied. However, it is not difficult to expect that many will have lost some, if not all, confidence in the medical system – a resource which they will need to obtain necessary support and help in their new circumstances.

Participating in a screening programme is generally seen as a responsible act, for example cervical smear testing programmes. As serum screening for fetal abnormality is more widely done, the anxiety it provokes at present may lessen. However, how individuals see risk is largely determined by how serious and difficult they feel the condition will be (Kerzin-Storrai, 1991). The concept of high and low risk is not only debatable at present, but it is fluid over time – there is evidence that some cases that genetic counsellors define as high risk today would not have been seen as such 20 years ago (Rothman, 1994). If a screening test does not pick up a large percentage of the condition screened for, it is not effective, but the more women screened, the more false positive results will be obtained. Who decides how many pregnant women will have the raised anxiety a false positive result produces, plus the trauma and risk of an invasive diagnostic test, in order to diagnose one abnormal fetus? (Green, 1990).

For the majority of women with a diagnosed fetal abnormality, the only choice is between termination, or continuing with the pregnancy. This raises the question of very many value judgements for the parents, with a frighteningly tragic decision to be made in a very short period of time. Society's values are extremely confusing, with a termination for fetal abnormality regarded with approval, but the life of a handicapped neonate, of perhaps virtually the same gestation, sacrosanct.

The growing ability to accurately diagnose fetal abnormality, and the resulting increased termination rate, may have many long-term effects on society as a whole, one being that with fewer abnormal babies born, the interest in exploring the causes of congenital abnormality may be reduced and therefore potentially dangerous environmental conditions (and drugs) may not be discovered.

The increased ease of access to antenatal diagnosis and termination reinforces the negative attitudes of society towards handicap and may reduce facilities and resources available for this vulnerable population even further.

Some parents may have other choices possible following the diagnosis of specific fetal abnormalities, and they may benefit from the increased availability of medical and surgical treatment, both before and after birth. This group of people will increase as resources, knowledge and experience grows in this area.

There are many other ethical issues surrounding fetal assessment. Informed choice is a particularly difficult subject, as the outcome of so much of fetal assessment is not able to be easily predicted. There is evidence that counselling before the 'routine' anomaly scan is inadequate (Smith and Marteau, 1995). Some women carrying an abnormal fetus do not wish to know, and would not contemplate termination – it is too late to try and meet their needs after a routine scan shows an abnormality.

Many results cannot predict the effects of the abnormality diagnosed (for example sex chromosome trisomy) [Garrett and Carlton, 1994], so the choice the parents make is not able to be 'informed'.

To be confident that they are making an informed choice, parents look to professionals for information. Recent media publicity concerning women who were diagnosed with a dead fetus and recommended for a surgical evacuation of retained products of conception, and subsequently found to have a viable pregnancy, calls all professional diagnoses into question. This is a field where there is no room for errors.

The disclosure of hereditary disorders discovered during antenatal diagnosis, to other members of the family, will break confidentiality with the client, and is a dilemma to be faced by the clinician if the client requests secrecy. As research into genetics progresses, the ability to diagnose carrier states and genetic propensity towards various conditions in the fetus is becoming possible. The ethics of breaching confidentiality also arises when considering how or when (or if) to make information about future disability available to the child, especially when in the USA 'wrongful life' legal cases have involved the damaged child/adult suing parents and clinicians (Harris, 1991). Also in the USA there have been cases of court-ordered caesarean sections against the mother's wishes, for the potential benefit of the fetus, as well as drug abusing mothers jailed for 'supplying drugs to a minor' via the umbilical cord. These cases raise the question of social control of pregnancy through assessment of the fetus and its perceived needs.

The future of fetal assessment has seemingly endless boundaries. As progress is made in gene mapping and technology, it is easy to see that there will one day be the ability to diagnose all fetal cytogenetic or Mendelian disorders by tests on fetal cells in maternal blood (Shulman and Elias, 1993). Gene therapy, a rapidly expanding field, if done for the fetus should in theory be more successful than if done at birth (when 90 per cent of adult cells are already present) [Evans et al, 1993].

Pre-implantation testing is already in use for those couples undergoing in vitro fertilization. If the success rates for IVF improve this may be an alternative to repeated terminations after antenatal diagnosis for those couples with a hereditary risk of abnormalities.

It is unlikely the future will show any reduction in new procedures and techniques in the field of fetal assessment, and many couples will achieve a healthy pregnancy and normal baby through these developments. However there is no doubt that the increase in testing will result in a greater need by parents for support and information from their midwife.

References

Alexander, S., Standwell-Smith, R., Buekens, P., Keirse, M. (1989). 'Biochemical assessment of fetal wellbeing'. In: Chalmers, I., Enkins, M., Keirse, M. (Eds). *Effective Care in Pregnancy and Childbirth.* Chapter 29. Oxford: Oxford University Press.

Alfirevic, Z., Neilson, J. (1993). 'Fetal growth retardation: methods of detection'. *Current Obstetrics and Gynaecology.* Vol.3, No.4, December pp.190-195.

Alfirevic, Z., Walkinshaw, S. (1994). 'Management of post-term pregnancy: to induce or not?' *British Journal of Hospital Medicine.* Vol.52, No.5, pp.218-221.

Annis, L. (1978). *The Child Before Birth.* New York: Cornell University Press.

Anteby, E., Tadmor, O., Revel, A., Yagel, S. (1994). 'Post-term pregnancies with normal cardiotocographs and amniotic fluid columns: the role of doppler evaluation in predicting perinatal outcomes'. *European Journal of Obstetrics, Gynaecology and Reproductive Biology.* Vol.54, No.2, April pp.93-98.

Arabin, B., Ragosch, V., Mohnhaupt, A. (1995). 'From biochemical to biophysical placental function tests in fetal surveillance'. *American Journal of Perinatology.* Vol.12, No.3, May pp.168-171.

Ault, K., Faro, S. (1993). 'Viruses, bacteria and protozoans in pregnancy: a sample of each' *Clinical Obstetrics and Gynecology* Vol.36, No.4, December pp.878-885.

Ballantyne, J. (1901). 'A plea for pro-mat hospitals' *British Medical Journal* Vol.1, 6th April pp.813-814.

Barker, D. (1993). 'Intrauterine growth retardation and adult disease' *Current Obstetrics and Gynaecology* Vol.3, No.4, December pp.200-206.

Bekedam, D. et al (1987). 'Heart rate variation and movement incidence in growth-retarded fetuses: the significance of antenatal late heart rate decelerations' *American Journal of Obstetrics and Gynaecology* Vol.157, pp.126-133.

Bennett, M., Little, G., Dewhurst, J., Chamberlain, G. (1982). 'Predictive values of ultrasound measurement in early pregnancy: a randomized control trial' *British Journal of Obstetrics and Gynaecology* Vol.89, May pp.338-341.

Bennett, P. (1988). 'Prostaglandins, preterm labour and infection' In: Chamberlain, G. (Ed). *Contemporary Obstetrics and Gynaecology.* London: Butterworth.

Berrebi, A. et al (1994). 'Termination of pregnancy for maternal toxoplasmosis' *Lancet* Vol.344, No.8914, 2nd July pp.34-39.

Best, J., Banatvala, J. (1990). 'Congenital virus infections' *British Medical Journal* Vol.300, 5th May pp.1151-1152.

Birth (1992). *News Section.* Vol.19, No.1, March p.42.

Blair, E., Stanley, F. (1988). 'Intrapartum asphyxia: a rare cause of cerebral palsy' *Journal of Pediatrics* Vol.12, pp.515-519.

Campbell, S. et al (1982). 'Short term psychological effect of early ultrasound scanning in pregnancy' *Journal of Psychomatic Obstetrics and Gynaecology*. Vol.1 pp.57-62.

Catanzarite, V. (1993). 'Amnioinfusion in the evaluation of severe oligohydramnios' *Perinatal Press* Vol.15, No.2, pp.25-26.

Challis, D., Trudinger, B. (1994). 'Doppler fetal assessment' *Current Obstetrics and Gynaecology* Vol.4, No.4, December pp.204-209.

Chamberlain, G. (1990). 'What is modern antenatal care of the fetus?' In: Chamberlain, G. (Ed). *Modern Antenatal Care of the Fetus* Oxford: Blackwell Scientific Publications.

Chard, T., Macintosh, M. (1992). 'Antenatal diagnosis of congenital abnormalities' In: Chard, T., Richards, M. (Eds). *Obstetrics in the 1990s: Current Controversies.* Oxford: MacKeith Press.

Chauhan, S. et al (1994). 'Estimate of birthweight among post-term pregnancy: clinical versus sonographic' *Journal of Maternal-Fetal Medicine* Vol.3 No.5 Sept/Oct pp.208-211.

Chervenak, F. (1992). 'Fetal blood sampling' In: Druzin, M. (Ed). *Antepartum Fetal Assessment.* Boston: Blackwell Scientific Publications.

Clapp, J. (1989). 'Physiological adaptation in fetal growth retardation' In: Spencer, J. (Ed). *Fetal Monitoring* Chapter 3. Kent: Castle House Publications Ltd.

Connor, E. et al (1994). 'Reduction of maternal-infant transmission of human immunodeficiency virus type 1 with zidovudine treatment' *New England Journal of Medicine* Vol.331, No.18, 3rd November pp.1173-1180.

Cuckle, H. et al (1990). 'Measurement of activity of urea resistant neutrophil alkaline phosphatase as an antenatal screening test for Down's Syndrome' *British Medical Journal* Vol.301, 3rd November pp.93-98.

Daker, M., Borrow, M. (1989). 'Screening for genetic disease and fetal anomaly during pregnancy' In: Chalmers, I., Enkins, M., Keirse, M. (Eds). *Effective Care in Pregnancy and Childbirth* Chapter 23. Oxford: Oxford University Press.

Dawes, M., Grudzinskas, J. (1991). 'Weighing does not help to find small babies' *British Journal of Obstetrics and Gynaecology* Vol.98, No.2, February pp.195-201.

Department of Health (1992). 'Women advised to take folic acid to reduce the risk of spina bifida babies' *Department of Health Press Release* H92/461 17th Dec.

Donner, C. et al. (1994). 'Accuracy of amniotic fluid testing before 21 weeks gestation in prenatal diagnosis of congenital CMV infection' *Prenatal Diagnosis* Vol.14, No.1, November pp.1055-1059.

Dornan, J., Harper, A. (1994). 'Where are we with doppler?' *British Journal of Obstetrics and Gynaecology.* Vol.101, No.3, March pp.190-191.

Droste, S. (1993). 'Genetic risk assessment in pregnancy' In: FitzSimmons, J. (Ed). *Prenatal Diagnosis.* Chapter One. New York: Elsevier.

Druzin, M. (1992). 'The non-stress test and contraction stress test' In: Druzin, M. (Ed). *Antepartum Fetal Assessment* Chapter 1 Boston: Blackwell Scientific Publications.

Dryden, R. (1978). *Before Birth.* London: Heinemann Education Books.

Dunn, D. et al. (1994). 'Mode of delivery and vertical transmission of HIV-1: a review of prospective studies' *Journal of Acquired Immune Deficiency Syndromes* Vol.7, No.10, October pp.1064-1066.

Emery, A. (1973). *Introduction to Antenatal Diagnosis of Genetic Disease* Edinburgh: Churchill Livingstone.

Enders, G. et al. (1994). 'Consequences of varicella and herpes zoster in pregnancy: prospective study of 1739 cases' *Lancet* Vol.343, No.8912, 18th June pp.1548-1552.

Engstrom, J. (1988). 'Measurement of fundal height' *Journal of Obstetric, Gynecologic and Neonatal Nursing* Vol.17, No.3, May/June pp.172-178.

Engstrom, J., McFarlin, B., Sampson, M. (1993). 'Fundal height measurement. Part 4 - accuracy of clinicians identification of the uterine fundus during pregnancy' *Journal of Nurse-Midwifery* Vol.38, No.6, Nov/Dec pp.318-323.

Engstrom, J., Ostrenga, K., Plass, R. (1989). 'The effect of maternal bladder volume on fundal height measurements'. *British Journal of Obstetrics and Gynaecology* Vol.96, No.8, August pp.987-991.

Engstrom, J., Sittler, C., Swift, K. (1994). 'Fundal height measurement. Part 5 - the effect of clinician bias on fundal height measurements' *Journal of Nurse-Midwifery* Vol.39, No.3, May/June pp.130-141.

Evans, M. (1993). 'Prenatal diagnosis in the future II: fetal therapy' In: FitzSimmons, J. (Ed). *Prenatal Diagnosis.* Chapter 10. New York: Elsevier.

Evans, M. et al. (1993). 'Efficacy of transabdominal multifetal pregnancy reduction: collaborative experience among the world's largest centers' *Obstetrics and Gynecology* Vol.82, No.1, pp.60-66.

Farr, A. (1988). *Dictionary of Medical Laboratory Sciences.* Oxford: Blackwell Scientific Publications.

Harris, J. (1991). 'Ethical aspects of prenatal diagnosis' In: Drife, J., Donnae, D. (Eds) *Antenatal Diagnosis of Fetal Abnormality.* Chapter 21 London: Springer-Verlag.

Firth, H. et al. (1994). 'Analysis of limb reduction defects in babies exposed to chorionic villus sampling' *Lancet* Vol.343, No.8905, 30th April pp.1069-1071.

Fisk, N., Rodeck, C. (1989). 'Antenatal diagnostic procedures' In: Spencer, J. (Ed). *Fetal Monitoring* Chapter 9. Kent: Castle House Publications Ltd.

Fisk, N., Rodeck, C. (1990). 'Detection of congenital abnormalities of the renal and urinary tract by ultrasound' In: Chamberlain, G. (Ed). *Modern Antenatal Care of the Fetus* Chapter 19. Oxford; Blackwell Scientific Publications.

Fox, H. (1991). 'A contemporary view of the human placenta' *Midwifery* Vol.7 pp.31-39.

Gabbe, S. (1986). 'Antepartum fetal assessment' In: Gabbe, S., Neibyl, J., Simpson, J. (Eds). *Obstetrics: Normal and Problem Pregnancies* Chapter 10. New York: Churchill Livingstone.

Garrett, C., Carlton, L. (1994). 'Difficult decisions in prenatal diagnosis' In: Abramsky, L., Chapple, J. (Eds). *Prenatal Diagnosis: The Human Side.* Chapter 6. London: Chapman & Hall.

Gibb, D., Greenough, A. (1991). 'Problems of multiple pregnancies' *British Journal of Hospital Medicine* Vol.46, December pp.376-370.

Gilbert, G. (1993). 'Chickenpox during pregnancy' *British Medical Journal* Vol.306, No.6885, 24th April pp.1079-1080.

Giorlandino, C., Bilancioni, E., D'Al Essio, P., Muzii, L. (1994). 'Risk of iatrogenic fetal infection at prenatal diagnosis' *Lancet* Vol.343, No.8902, 9th April pp.922-923.

Gosden, C., Nicolaides, K., Whitting, V. (1994). *Is My Baby Alright: A Guide for Expectant Parents*. Oxford: Oxford University Press.

Grandjean, H., Sarramon, M. (1995). 'Sonographic measurement of nuchal skinfold thickness for detection of Down Syndrome in the second-trimester fetus: a multicenter prospective study' *Obstetrics and Gynecology* Vol.85, No.1, January pp.103-106.

Green, J., Statham, H. (1993). 'Testing for fetal abnormality in routine antenatal care' *Midwifery* Vol.9, No.3, September pp.124-136.

Green, J. (1990). 'Prenatal screening and diagnosis: some psychological and social issues' *British Journal of Obstetrics and Gynaecology* Vol.97, No.12, December pp.1074-1076.

Green, J., Statham, H., Snowdon, C. (1992). 'Screening for fetal abnormality: attitudes and experience' In: Chard, T., Richards, M. (Eds). *Obstetrics in the 1990s: Current Controversies*. Chapter 5. Oxford: MacKeith Press.

Griffiths, P. D. (1991). 'Virology' In: Phillips, E., Setchell, M. (Eds). *Scientific Foundations of Obstetrics and Gynaecology*. 4th edition. London: Butterworth/Heinemann.

Grudzinskas, J., Westergaard, J., Teisner, B. (1986). 'Biochemical assessment of placental function' *Clinical Obstetrics and Gynaecology* Vol.13 pp.553-569.

Hackett, G., Nicolaides, K., Campbell, S. (1987). 'Doppler ultrasound assessment of fetal and uteroplacental circulations in severe second trimester oligohydamnios' *British Journal of Obstetrics and Gynaecology* Vol.94 November pp.1074-77.

Hadlock, et al. (1985). 'Estimation of fetal weight with the use of head, body and femur measurements - a prospective study'. *American Journal of Obstetrics and Gynecology* Vol.151 pp.333-337.

Hamner, L. et al (1993). 'Efficacy and safety of fetal acoustic stimulation testing' *Journal of Maternal-Fetal Investigation* Vol.3, No.2, pp.113-116.

Hanretty, K., Neilson, J., Fleming, J. (1990). 'Re-evaluation of clinical estimation of fetal weight. A comparison with ultrasound' *Journal of Obstetrics and Gynaecology* Vol.10, No.3, Jan pp.199-201.

Harper, P. (1981). *Practical Genetic Counselling*. Bristol: John Wright & Sons Ltd.

Harris, J. (1991). 'Ethical aspects of prenatal diagnosis'. In Drife, J., Donnai, D. (Eds). *Antenatal Diagnosis of Fetal Abnormalities*. London: Springer Verlag.

Hedegaard, et al (1993). 'Psychological distress in pregnancy and preterm delivery' *British Medical Journal* Vol.307, No.6898, 24th July pp.234-239.

Hepburn, M., Rosenburg, K. (1986). 'An audit of the detection and management of small-for-gestational age babies' *British Journal of Obstetrics and Gynaecology* Vol.93 March pp.212-216.

Hohlfield, P. et al (1994). 'Prenatal diagnosis of congenital toxoplasmosis with a polymerase-chain-reaction test on amniotic fluid'. *New England Journal of Medicine* Vol.331, No.11, 15th Sept. pp.695-699.

Horner, P., Goldmeier, D. (1989). 'Antenatal screening for syphilis'. *British Medical Journal* Vol.299, 30th Sept p.859.

Huisjes, H. et al (1980). 'Obstetrical - neonatal neurological relationships. A replication study.' *European Journal of Gynaecological Reproductive Biology* Vol. 10 pp.247-256.

Hurley, R. (1991). 'Virology' In: Phillips, E., Setchell, M. (Eds). *Scientific Foundations of Obstetrics and Gynaecology* 4th edition. London: Butterworth/Heinemann.

Hytten, F. (1984). 'The effect of work on placental function and fetal' In: Chamberlain, G. (Ed). *Pregnancy, Women and Work* London: Royal Society of Medicine.

James, D. (1991). 'Limitations of fetal biophysical assessment' *Contemporary Review of Obstetrics & Gynaecology* Vol.3 pp.69-74.

James, D. (1993). 'Monitoring the biophysical profile' *British Journal of Hospital Medicine* Vol.49, No.8 pp.561-563.

Kenyon, S. (1994). 'Scanning in late pregnancy' *British Journal of Midwifery* Vol.2, No.2, February pp.51-55.

Kerzin-Storrai, L. (1991). 'Psychological aspects of genetic counselling'. *Research Trust for Metabolic Diseases in Children News* Vol.3, No.8, June pp.4-6.

Ko, T. et al (1995). 'Ultrasonographic scanning of placental thickness and the prenatal diagnosis of homozygous alpha-thalassaemia 1 in the second trimester' *Prenatal Diagnosis* Vol.15, No.1, January pp.7-10.

Kyle, P. et al (1994). 'Life without amniocentesis: elevated maternal serum a-fetoprotein in the Manitoba program 1986-91' *Ultrasound in Obstetrics and Gynecology* Vol.4, No.3, May pp.199-204.

Ladermacher, D., Vemeulen, R., Harter, J., Arts, N. (1981). 'Circumvallate placenta and congenital malformation' *Lancet* Vol.1, No. 8222, 28th March p.732.

Logan, S. (1990). 'Viral infections in pregnancy' In: Chamberlain, G. (Ed). *Modern Antenatal Care of the Fetus* Oxford: Blackwell Scientific Publications.

Low, J., Simpson, L., Ramsey, D. (1992). 'The clinical diagnosis of asphyxia responsible for brain damage in the human fetus' *American Journal of Obstetrics & Gynecology* Vol.167, No.1, July pp.11-15.

MacGregor, E. (1991). 'Dilemmas in genetic screening' *Nursing* Vol.4, No.41, 12th September pp.13-14.

Marteau, T. et al (1992). 'Psychological effects of false positive results in prenatal screening for fetal abnormality: a prospective study' *Prenatal Diagnosis* Vol.12 pp.205-214.

Martinez, F. et al (1994). 'The effect of paternal smoking on the birthweight of newborns whose mothers did not smoke' *American Journal of Public Health* Vol.84, No.9, September pp.1489-1491.

Mastroiacovo, P. et al (1993). 'Transverse limb reduction defects after chorion villus sampling: a retrospective cohort study' *Prenatal Diagnosis* Vol.13, No.11, November pp.1051-1056.

McDonald, H. et al (1992). 'Prenatal microbiological risk factors associated with preterm birth' *British Journal of Obstetrics and Gynaecology* Vol.99, No.3, March pp.190-196.

McGregor, J., French, J., Sen, K. (1991). 'Antimicrobial therapy in preterm premature rupture of membranes: results of a prospective, double-blind, placebo-controlled trial of erythromycin' *American Journal of Obstetrics & Gynaecology* Vol.164, No.3, September pp.632-640.

McParland, P., Johnson, H. (1993). 'Time to reinvent the wheel' *British Journal of Obstetrics and Gynaecology* Vol.100, No.11, Nov pp.1061-1062.

McParland, P., Pearce, M. (1990). 'Uteroplacental and fetal blood flow' In: Chamberlain, G. (Ed). *Modern Antenatal Care of the Fetus* Chapter 6 Oxford: Blackwell Scientific Publications.

Meisner, L. (1993). 'Laboratory procedures and quality assurance in prenatal cytogenetic analysis' In: FitzSimmons, J. (Ed). *Prenatal Diagnosis* Chapter 7 New York: Elsevier.

Miller, E. (1990). 'Rubella infection in pregnancy' In: Chamberlain, G. (Ed). *Modern Antenatal Care of the Fetus* Chapter 13 Oxford: Blackwell Scientific Publications.

Mohide, P., Keirse, M. (1989). 'Biophysical assessment of fetal wellbeing' In: Chalmers, I., Enkins, M., Keirse, M. (Eds). *Effective Care in Pregnancy and Childbirth* Chapter 13. Oxford: Oxford University Press.

Murphy, K. et al (1990). 'Birth asphyxia and the intrapartum cardiotocograph' *British Journal of Obstetrics and Gynaecology* Vol.97, No.6, June pp.470-479.

Mutale, T. et al (1991). 'Life events and low birthweight - analysis by infants preterm and small for gestational age' *British Journal of Obstetrics and Gynaecology* Vol.98, No.2, February pp.166-172.

Neilson, J. (1990). 'The measurement of fetal growth'. In: Chamberlain, G. (Ed). *Modern Antenatal Care of the Fetus* Chapter 5. Oxford: Blackwell Scientific Publications.

Newburn, M. (1993). 'The triple test - what do you think?' *New Generation* Vol.12, No.3, September pp.43-44.

Nicholaides, K., Bilardo, C., Soothill, P., Campbell, S. (1988). 'Absence of end dystolic frequency in umbilical arteries: a sign of fetal hypoxia' *British Medical Journal* Vol.297, No.6655, 22nd October pp.1026-27.

Nicolaides, K., Economides, D. (1990). 'Cordocentesis in the investigation of small-for-gestational age fetuses' In: Chamberlain, G. (Ed). *Modern Antenatal Care of the Fetus* Chapter 7. Oxford: Blackwell Scientific Publications.

Nicolini, U. et al (1994). 'Prenatal diagnosis of congenital human cytomegalovirus infection' *Prenatal Diagnosis* Vol.14, No.10, Oct pp.903-906.

Nijhuis, J. (1989). 'Fetal behavioural states' In: Spencer, J. (Ed). *Fetal Monitoring* Chapter 5. Kent: Castle House Publications Ltd.

O'Callaghan, et al. (1992). 'Risk of schizophrenia in adults born after obstetric complications and their association with early onset of illness: a controlled study' *British Medical Journal* Vol.305, No.6864, 21st November pp.1256-1259.

Obiekwe, B., Chard, T. (1983). 'A comparative study of the clinical use of four placenta proteins in the third trimester' *Journal of Perinatal Medicine* Vol.11 pp.121-126.

Oepkes, D. et al (1994). 'The use of ultrasonography and doppler in the prediction of fetal haemolytic anaemia: a multivariate analysis' *British Journal of Obstetrics and Gynaecology* Vol.101, No.8, August pp.680-684.

Patrick, J. et al (1982). 'Patterns of gross fetal body movements over 24-hour observation intervals during the last 10 weeks of pregnancy' *American Journal of Obstetrics & Gynecology* Vol.142, No.4, pp.363-371.

Peacock, J. et al (1991). 'Cigarette smoking and birthweight: type of cigarette smoked and a possible threshold effect' *International Journal of Epidemiology* Vol.20, No.2, June pp.405-412.

Pearce, J., Campbell, C. (1987). 'A comparison of symphis-fundal height and ultrasound as screening for light-for-gestational age infants' *British Journal of Obstetrics & Gynaecology* Vol.94, February pp.100-104.

Pearce, J. (1990). 'The ultrasound diagnosis of neural tube defects' In: Chamberlain, G. (Ed) *Modern Antenatal Care of the Fetus* Chapter 17 Oxford: Blackwell Scientific Publications.

Pillai, M., James, D. (1990a). 'The development of fetal heart rate patterns during normal pregnancy' *Obstetrics & Gynecology* Vol.76 pp.812-816.

Pillai, M., James, D. (1990b). 'Hiccups and breathing in the human fetus' *Archives of Diseases of Childhood* Vol.65 pp.1072-75.

Pinette, M. et al (1989). 'Maternal smoking and accelerated placental maturation' *Obstetrics & Gynecology* Vol.73, No.3 (part 1) March pp.379-382.

Proud, J. (1989). 'Placental grading' In: Robinson, S., Thomson, A. (Eds). *Midwives, Research and Childbirth* Vol.1 Chapter 5. London: Chapman and Hall.

Proud, J. (1994). *Understanding Obstetric Ultrasound: A Guide for Midwives and other Health Professionals*. Cheshire: Books for Midwives Press.

Public Health Laboratory Service Working Party of Fifth Disease (1990). 'Prospective study of human parvovirus (B19) infection in pregnancy' *British Medical Journal* Vol.300, 5th May, pp.1166-1170.

Richardson, B. (1989). 'Fetal breathing movements' In: Spencer, J. (Ed). *Fetal Monitoring* Chapter 12. Kent: Castle House Publications Ltd.

Ridgway, G. (1990). 'Bacterial infections of the fetus and newborn' In: Chamberlain, G. (Ed). *Modern Antenatal Care of the Fetus* Chapter 11 Oxford: Blackwell Scientific Publications.

Rogers, M., Chan, E., Ho, A. (1992). 'Fundal height: does prior knowledge of gestational age influence the measurement?' *Journal of Obstetrics and Gynaecology* Vol.12, No.1, January pp.4-5.

Rona, R., Gulliford, M., Chinn, S. (1993). 'Effects of prematurity and intrauterine growth on respiratory health and lung function in childhood' *British Medical Journal* Vol.306, No.6881, 27th March pp.817-820.

Rothman, B. (1994). *The Tentative Pregnancy: Amniocentesis and the Sexual Politics of Motherhood*. 2nd edition. London: Pandora.

Rowson, K., Rees, T., Mahy, B. (1981). *A Dictionary of Virology*. Oxford: Blackwell Scientific Publications.

Royal College of Obstetrics and Gynaecology (1984). *Report of the Working Party on Routine Ultrasound Examination in Pregnancy.* London: RCOG.

Royburst, M., Seidman, D. (1990). 'Fundal height - can we trust the umbilicus?' *Lancet* Vol.338, No.8771, 5th October pp.891-892.

Ryder, R. et al (1989). 'Ethical aspects of prenatal diagnosis' In: Drife, J., Donnai, D. (Eds) *Antenatal Diagnosis of Fetal Abnormality.* Chapter 21 London: Springer-Verlag.

Saunders, N., Paterson, C. (1991). 'Can we abandon Naegele's rule?' *Lancet* Vol.337, No.8741, 9th March pp.600-601.

Sharif, K., Whittle, M. (1993). 'Routine antenatal fetal heart rate auscultation: is it necessary?' *Journal of Obstetrics & Gynaecology* Vol.13, No.2, March pp.111-113.

Sharland, G., Allan, L. (1990). 'Detection of congenital abnormalities of the cardiovascular system by ultrasound' In: Chamberlain, G. (Ed). *Modern Antenatal Care of the Fetus* Chapter 18. Oxford: Blackwell Scientific Publications.

Shulman, L., Elias, S. (1993). 'Prenatal diagnosis in the future I: new diagnostic modalities' In: Fitzsimmons, J. (Ed). *Prenatal Diagnosis* New York: Elsevier.

Simpson, J. (1986). 'Genetic counselling and prenatal diagnosis' In: Gabbe, S., Niebyl, J., Simpson, J. (Eds). *Obstetrics: Normal and Problem Pregnancies* Chapter 8 New York: Churchill Livingstone.

Smith, D., Marteau, T. (1995). 'Detecting fetal abnormality: serum screening and fetal anomaly scans' *British Journal of Midwifery* Vol.3, No.3, March pp.133-136.

Spencer, J. (1989). 'Screening and diagnosis and fetal growth retardation' In: Spencer, J. (Ed). *Fetal Monitoring* Kent: Castle House Publications Ltd.

Spencer, J. (1990). 'Antepartum cardiotocography' In: Chamberlain, G. (Ed). *Modern Antenatal Care of the Fetus* Chapter 9 Oxford: Blackwell Scientific Publications.

Steer, P. (1990). 'What determines fetal heart rate?' In: Chamberlain, G. (Ed). *Modern Antenatal Care of the Fetus* Chapter 8 Oxford: Blackwell Scientific Publications.

Stirrat, G. (1991). 'The immunological system' In: Hytten, F., Chamberlain, G. (Eds). *Clinical Physiology in Obsterics.* Oxford: Blackwell Scientific Publications.

Stray-Pedersen, B. (1993). 'New aspect of perinatal infections' *Annals of Medicine* Vol.25, No.3, June pp.295-300.

Stuart, J. et al (1989). 'Symphysis-fundus measurements in screening for small-for-dates infants: a community based study in Gloucestershire' *Journal of the Royal College of General Practitioners* Vol.39, No.319, Feb pp.45-48.

Tanner, J. (1989). *Foetus Into Man: Physical Growth from Conception to Maturity* 2nd edition. p.119. Ware: Castlemead Publications.

Taylor, D. (1989). 'Neurological sequelae of intrauterine deprivation' In: Spencer, J. (Ed). *Fetal Monitoring.* Chapter 4. Kent: Castle House Publications Ltd.

Teitelman, A. et al. (1990). 'Effect of maternal work activity on preterm birth and low birth weight' *American Journal of Epidemiology* Vol.131, No.3, March pp.131-133.

Terry, G. et al. (1986). 'First trimester prenatal diagnosis of congenital rubella: a laboratory investigation' *British Medical Journal* Vol.292, No.6525, 5th April pp.930-933.

Trudinger, B., Giles, W., Cook, R. (1985). 'Flow velocity waveforms in the maternal uteroplacental and fetal umbilical placental circulations' *British Journal of Obstetrics and Gynaecolgy* Vol.152 No.2 p.152.

Tsang, H., Manning, F. (1992). 'Fetal biophysical profile scoring' In: Druzin, M.L. (Ed). *Antepartum Fetal Assessment* Chapter 3. Boston: Blackwell Scientific Publications.

Visser, G. et al. (1989). 'Vibro-acoustic stimulation of the human fetus: effect on behavioural state organization' *Early Human Development* Vol.19 pp.285-296.

Wadhwa, P. et al. (1993). 'The association between prenatal stress and infant birth weight and gestational age at birth: a prospective investigation' *American Journal of Obstetrics and Gynecology* Vol.169, No.4, October pp.858-865.

Wagner, W. (1992). 'Intrauterine growth retardation' In: Druzin, M. L. (Ed). *Antepartum Fetal Assessment* Chapter 15. Boston: Blackwell Scientific Publications.

Wald, N. et al. (1994). 'Four-marker serum screening for Down's Syndrome'. *Prenatal Diagnosis* Vol.14, No.8, August pp.707-716.

Wald, N., Kennard, A., Densem, J. (1992). 'Antenatal maternal serum screening for Down's Syndrome: results of a demonstration project' *British Medical Journal* Vol.305, No.6850, 15th August pp.391-39

Wang, F., Smaill, F. (1989). 'Infection in pregnancy' In: Chalmers, I., Enkins, M., Keirse, M. (Eds). *Effective Care in Pregnancy and Childbirth* Oxford: Oxford University Press.

Wapner, R., Johnson, A., Abbott, J. (1993). 'Invasive methods of prenatal diagnosis: amniocentesis, CVS and cordocentesis' In: FitzSimmons, J. (Ed). *Prenatal Diagnosis* Chapter 4. New York: Elsevier.

Warren, R. (1990). 'Chorion villus sampling' In: Chamberlain, G. (Ed). *Modern Antenatal Care of the Fetus* Chapter 15. Oxford: Blackwell Scientific Publications.

Watts, D. (1993). 'Infection and fetal development' In: FitzSimmons, J. (Ed). *Prenatal Diagnosis* Chapter 3. New York: Elsevier.

Westergaard, J. et al. (1985). 'Does ultrasound examination render biochemical tests obsolete in the prediction of early pregnancy failure?' *British Journal of Obstetrics and Gynaecology* Vol.92, January pp.77-83.

Wheeler, T. (1991). 'Cardiotocography' In: Phillip, E., Setchell, M. (Eds). *Scientific Foundations of Obstetrics and Gynaecology* 4th edition. Chapter 53 London: Butterworth/Heinemann.

Wolf, H., Oosting, H., Treffers, P. (1989). 'A longitudinal study of the relationship between placental and fetal growth as measured by ultrasonography' *American Journal of Obstetrics and Gynecology* Vol.161, No.5, November pp.1140-1146.

Youssef, A. et al. (1993). 'Superiority of amniotic fluid index over amniotic fluid pocket measurement for predicting bad fetal outcome' *Southern Medical Journal* Vol.86, No.4, April pp.426-429.

Index

Books for Midwives Press

Books for Midwives Press publish books written by experts in the midwifery field to meet the practical needs of the working midwife and midwifery students. Below is a list of our current titles.

MIRIAD (2nd edition)	McCormick and Renfrew	£17.95
Midwives and Management	Rosemary Cross	£12.95
Relaxation and Exercise for the Childbearing Year	Brayshaw and Wright	£5.95
Electronic Monitoring of the Fetal Heart	Williams and Blanchard	£9.95
Breastfeeding: A Guide for Midwives	Henschel and Inch	£9.95
Gynaecology for Everywoman	Philip Rhodes	£9.95
Listen with Mother	Maternity Alliance	£9.95
The Pregnant Drug Addict	Catherine Siney	£9.95
Waterbirth	Dianne Garland	£10.95
Super-Vision	ARM	£9.95
A Short History of Clinical Midwifery	Philip Rhodes	£17.95
Communicating Midwifery	Caroline Flint	£12.95
Midwives and 'Changing Childbirth'	Walton and Hamilton	£9.95
Legal Aspects of Midwifery	Bridgit Dimond	£14.95
Sexuality and Motherhood	Irene Walton	£10.95
Reactions to Motherhood	Jean Ball	£10.95
Holding On?	Hazel McHaffie	£9.95
Aquanatal Exercises	Gillian Halksworth	£6.95
MIRIAD	NPEU	£14.95
Understanding Obstetric Ultrasound	Jean Proud	£10.95
Antenatal Investigations (Revised)	Maureen Boyle	£6.95
HIV Infection in Pregnancy	Caroline Shepherd	£6.95
Teaching Physical Skills for the Childbearing Year	Brayshaw and Wright	£10.95

If you would like to receive details about future titles and be placed on our mailing list, please send your name, address and telephone number to the address given below.

Please order *Books for Midwives Press* titles from your usual bookseller and encourage them to stock midwifery titles. If you prefer you can order directly from us by sending a cheque (made payable to Books for Midwives Press) or by telephoning our hotline on 0161 929 0929 for credit/debit card orders (Access/Visa/Switch/Delta).

For overseas postage please add 25% of the total price. All UK orders are sent postage free.

Please send orders or requests for catalogues/information to:

BOOKS FOR MIDWIVES PRESS
Freepost WA1836
Hale
Cheshire
WA15 9BR

0161 929 0929